Cancer Can Be Cured!

Father Romano Zago, OFM
(Order of Friars Minor)

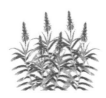

Part of the profits from the sale of this book will be allocated to the charity works of Father Romano Zago in Brazil.

The book in Italian, "Di Cancro si può Guarire," was translated by AL NABER Traduzioni

On the cover: Aloe arborescens plant in the garden of the Sanctuary of the Agony of Jesus (olive grove), Gethsemane, Jerusalem, Israel.

Photograph: Fray Delfin Fernandex Taboarda, OFM

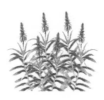

Senior Editor, B4Deadline
Janet Musick

Assistant Editor, B4Deadline
Cathy Musick

Cover and Interior Design
Just Ink

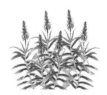

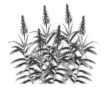

Cancer Can Be Cured!

This small book teaches how to treat cancer and other diseases, practically and inexpensively, without being subjected to mutilation or using pharmaceutical drugs, without side effects, and without having to leave home. – Father Romano Zago

Father Romano Zago, OFM, was born in Lajeado (RS) Brazil on August 11, 1932. He was ordained a Franciscan Friar in 1958 after having studied philosophy and theology. In 1971, he received a degree in literature and foreign languages (Latin, Portuguese, French and Spanish) from the faculty of literature at Pontifical Catholic University of Rio Grande do Sul.

In 1988, while presiding at the San Antonio parish in Pouso Novo (RS) Brazil, he learned from local natives about a potent all-natural Aloe arborescens recipe they use for curing cancer. He began to test it with the chronically ill. It was here he first observed the positive results obtained with nutrition against advanced disease states. Afterwards, he was sent to Jerusalem and Italy, where he continued to see great success in the chronically ill being cured when he recommended they try this recipe made with the whole leaf of the native Aloe arborescens plant. This inspired him to devote his life to research and education on Aloe and the recipe that has been published in three books he has written. At the request of many people and organizations, he has given lectures and conferences in Portugal, Spain, Switzerland, France, Italy and Brazil about the

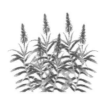

ability of the human body to heal and regulate itself when supplied with the cell-required concentrated micronutrients found in the polysaccharides (complex sugar molecules) of this Aloe plant species and the recipe.

"Aloe isn't medicine and yet...it Cures!" is another book by Father Romano Zago that continues the story of the Brazilian recipe with Aloe arborescens that is told in this book, "Cancer Can Be Cured," which includes an appendix titled "The Scientific Monographic History of Aloe Vera and Aloe Arborescens." In "Aloe isn't medicine and yet...it Cures", Father Zago explains how the abundant supply of herbal therapeutic and medicinal properties of Aloe arborescens restores the immune system so the cells and organs of the body can regain their normal functioning. He indicates, in simple practice, how to use the plant recipe to detoxify the whole body and boost the immune system to fight over 100 types of illnesses, including diabetes, depression and obesity.

> *Aloe arborescens is cultivated in regions of Brazil, Africa and the Mediterranean, but not North America.*

Contents

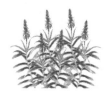

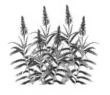

Introduction

After having heard of cancer being cured using the method explained in this book, many people have asked us to reveal the secret. The method we propose is contained in this work that I benevolently present to you to read.

I do not consider myself the creator of the recipe. Nor do I wish to appear as the pioneer, or the first to have used this recipe with positive results. This would not be true. Long before me, there were others who could claim this right.

This book is merely intended to publicize this method, which has proven effective on many occasions. If I have any credit, it is for having divulged it. What is written in these unpretentious pages is merely the record of a procedure that has given positive results, a procedure used by myself and others who know the recipe and use it with great success. Why not use the suggestions provided here in your case? The procedure is simple and easily available.

This recipe is inexpensive with no contraindications or negative side effects, targeted at alleviating the suffering of the sick and those directly or indirectly connected to them, who are sometimes helpless when faced with the enormity of the problem.

If some people have been cured using this simple and inexpensive method, why should we not offer the same opportunity to a great number of people? This is my goal.

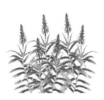

I do not profess to offer a magic method. But, because of the importance of this method, I do not wish to keep it a secret or use it only for my own benefit. That would be selfish.

The idea is to inform people of the existence of a recipe to cure cancer that has already been used, to offer a method accessible to all who are interested. The book explains how those who wish to can put this opportunity into practice.

Moreover, I do not intend to set aside the commendable medical class or, even worse, to discredit all scientific studies carried out to solve the problem of cancer, this plague of the century. All research performed in the battle against this disease is worthy of great praise, wherever it comes from. All that has already been done and is still to be done to finally solve the problem continues to be valid and deserves our full support and consideration. We hope that continual development of these investigations will allow man to dominate this disease that has long been a source of anguish for mankind. Let us help one another in this common war; it affects us all and must involve us all.

I wish to offer my modest collaboration to alleviate the atrocious suffering of man, so humiliated by the inevitability of surgical operations and those applications that disfigure him, this being the only treatment currently available in traditional medicine. I wish to spare those suffering from cancer from the dreadful consequences of radiotherapy, chemotherapy (a true assault on the body!) and other techniques of this nature. The system indicated here is a great deal cheaper, painless and natural. The human body heals itself, and nutrition derived from the Aloe arborescens plant provides the resources to accomplish the work.

People can use it from their own homes. The results are so satisfactory that people who have been healed, even those in the terminal phases of cancer, are able to return to their normal lives in two or three months, with even greater vigor and with a better quality of life, possibly because they are able to enjoy life once again after all had seemed irrevocably lost to them. I would like this recipe to be used along with all other methods, those already known and those still to be discovered, to form a united front to eliminate this fatal disease permanently from the face of the earth.

The purpose of this book, in its simplicity and clarity, is to provide a sign for those having to combat terrible illnesses such as cancer and other degenerative diseases.

Dear friend, if someone close to you has this dreadful disease and is undergoing the traditional treatments, offer them this simple method. It can work. It must work. It has caused true healing many, many times, saving lives. Oh, if there were only statistics on the healings that have taken place across the five continents! It costs nothing to try. You lose nothing. And a life can be saved.

Dear reader, it is my wish that, by following this simple, inexpensive, entirely natural method, without contraindications, you can restore your loved ones to health, allowing them to regain their full vitality, twice as joyfully, having seen the specter of imminent death, a death that seemed inevitable, fade away. You will feel the indescribable euphoria of having defeated something that seemed beyond your power. It will be as if you have given those who have been healed new life; you will have returned them to share life with the other living beings.

And within you will sing: "Blessed is God who gave man so many plants and herbs useful to combat disease, to allow life to continue, and continue in health!"

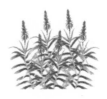

If you don't know Aloe (there are 300 to 400 classified varieties, and hundreds still to be classified or for which research has not been performed), choose the plant shown on the cover of this book – Aloe "arborescens." There are some twenty varieties of arborescens, which is the most widely diffused species in Brazil. When I mention Aloe, I am referring to the arborescens variety.

Dr. Aldo Facetti, phytology technician and herbalist, who interviewed me for more than an hour on "TV Riviera," transmitted in the areas of Massa, Viareggio, Lucca, Pisa and Carrara, guarantees that "Aloe vera or barbadensis" provides 40% of the active ingredients against cancer, while the arborescens variety provides 70%. For ease in finding and using the recipe, it is printed on the back cover.

Many people cannot possibly prepare the juice recipe fresh from home for various reasons and must rely on a commercial source for this 10-day liquid recipe supplied in a 16-oz. dark bottle. In this case, it is important to choose a manufacturer that uses premier-quality five-year old Aloe arborescens plants harvested at the proper time, processed by grinding the whole leaf into a juice without heating, cold pressing or freeze drying in order to retain all the active polysaccharides and phytonutrients needed to guarantee maximum effectiveness. Finally, the recipe must have at least 40% Aloe arborescens juice, honey, 1% alcohol and be stabilized for a long shelf life without the use of harmful preservatives.

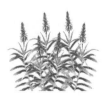

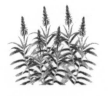

The Knowledge

After a day of work engrossed in a true kaleidoscope of activities aimed at covering various developing sectors of modern life, one after another the Friars Minor return home for dinner to recoup energy for a new day.

Absorbed in the habits of the Order, in the same way other citizens are absorbed in their own lives, after a regenerating shower the Franciscan sons of the earth from Rio Grande do Sul rest while sipping tea. While the small bowl of bitter tea is passed from hand to hand, according to tradition, a healthy conversation springs up covering a wide range of subjects: theology, philosophy, politics, parties, government, sociology, the parish, the Church, the Order, the province, ecumenicalism, the weather, the facts of the day, corruption, abortion, birth control, the third world, multinational companies, football, and so on.

On a day like many others, the ritual is repeated, although the subject being discussed this time is scientific development, its effects, and its amazing successes. The theme of the conversation touches on the fact, incredible but true, that large sums of money are currently allocated to establish funds or resources aimed at encouraging studies on curing cancer.

After various considerations on this subject, Father Arno Reckziegel appears. He is the new provincial father, appointed to this office after having worked in the parish on the outskirts

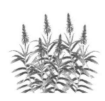

of the town. As if he were a magician taking an ace from his sleeve, he states that he has the solution to the problem, leaving the attentive audience flabbergasted.

"Of course, my friends, it is possible to cure cancer! This is why cancer is not a problem for the people from the suburbs. Or rather, it is a problem that has a solution."

"But how?" asks the most fascinated person in the group.

"Down in the shantytown in Rio Grande where I worked for a few years, every day I witnessed the healing of simple people with cancer," says Father Reckziegel. "I could quote the case of an elderly colored lady with skin cancer. After the cure, she is still living a normal life in her hut."

"But that's impossible!" one of the listeners says. "Did she truly have cancer?"

"Cancer found by medical tests. I quote the case of an unheard of humble person, but I could just as easily quote the healing of famous people who took the same treatment. We know of people of national fame who were healed of their disease with the same method used by the elderly lady from the suburbs of the Port City. The method heals people, whether they are poor and unheard of, or colored or famous, without discrimination. It works for everyone. Nature has no preferences. She answers all those who wish to take advantage of her."

"Listen, Brother, what is this magic recipe that heals cancer? Tell us without further delay, my friend, how the people of the suburbs down in Noiva-do-Mar cure tumors?"

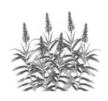

"I wish to emphasize there is no magic recipe whatsoever," Father Reckziegel says firmly. "It is very simple. Much simpler than one would imagine. Simple, cheap and natural. Unfortunately, almost no one knows of it and believes in it."

"If it is simple, cheap and natural, tells us about it immediately; I am eager to learn," an eager friar says. "The first day I hear of someone who is ill, I will recommend the magic recipe. I will be its greatest proponent so no one will need to die again from this terrible disease."

"I repeat, it is very simple. Everyone in the shantytown knows the recipe. No one there dies of cancer because the recipe is passed by word of mouth to anyone who is interested. Moreover, it is not secret. Only those who do not wish to live die of cancer in the shantytown. If this disease is diagnosed, everyone knows the answer. And everyone makes use of it."

"How wonderful! Dear God, tell us immediately about this blessed recipe! I've already said I can't wait to learn it."

"Here it is. Take note: half a kilogram of bees' honey, two Aloe leaves and three or four spoonfuls of distillate."

"Tell us more."

"There's nothing else to explain or add," Father Reckziegel tells his attentive audience. "That is the recipe. Remove the spines along the edge of the leaves and any dirt deposited by nature. Place the three ingredients – honey, Aloe and distillate – in the blender. Blend them well to obtain a light mixture and the mixture that cures cancer is ready."

"You must be joking! It's too simple to be true."

"But, my dear friend, I am extremely serious. This is by no means a joke. If you think I'm joking or pulling your leg, go and visit our shantytown in Rio Grande. You can ask the elderly colored lady, lovely lady even if humble, who was cured by this recipe."

"And how is this mixture taken?"

"One tablespoonful at breakfast time, one at lunch time, and another at dinner time. Always before meals, about 10, 20 or 30 minutes before. Shake the jar well before taking it. Keep it in the vegetable compartment of the fridge."

"But if this recipe is so miraculous, why is it not widely used? It should be announced throughout the world! Advertising space should be purchased in the mass media, in programs with the highest audiences, to disclose the discovery, so that no one else becomes the victim of this relentless disease."

"The recipe is truly as simple as this, but there are interests at play that prevent this extremely important discovery from being divulged or promoted. Cancer must continue to take lives. If the disease is cured, a rich source of earning will be lost. Cancer is a useful contraceptive to limit the number of poor people in the world and leave a larger slice of the cake on the table for the rich. Unfortunately, in Brazil, only the rich are able to afford lengthy, costly and sophisticated treatment. When the poor with their limited resources get cancer, they must die. These are the politics of those governing the planet."

The conversation is interrupted at this point as it is time for the community to recite Vespers, the afternoon prayer. However, one of the friars has learned the recipe by heart and heads toward the choir, observing the bell. But he has decided to divulge the recipe at any cost.

While the friars are in the choir reciting Vespers, the official Church prayer, Paolina is in the kitchen of the Provincialate preparing rare steak and onions which, together with rice grown locally and various types of salad and fruit, is the simple meal of the Friars Minor in Rio Grande do Sul. With her work, Paolina also performs her own liturgy which, in the same manner as the friars', rises harmoniously, like small psalms, to reach the presence of God.

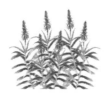

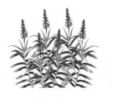

Putting the Knowledge into Practice

One day, while I was returning from a village chapel, the blacksmith stopped me.

"Father, you know my uncle Giovanni from Forqueta? He's got prostate cancer and is in the Marques de Sousa hospital. The doctor says there is no cure for his case. He tells us he only has a few days to live. Can I ask you on behalf of his family to perform extreme unction? Please go as soon as possible, as he is really sick."

"First, thank you for telling me. I will go and anoint him with the oil for the sick. How strange! I remember him well. I can still see him at Mass last month, in the first row on the left. I am shocked at the news you have given me today!"

"I'm afraid it's true, Father," the blacksmith said. "You know that the symptoms of this disease almost always appear when it is already at an advanced stage."

"Is your uncle conscious? Do you think I could wait until tomorrow to visit him?"

"Of course. The disease has made him very weak, but don't worry; he'll still be here tomorrow. However, the doctor says he will die before the end of the week. I have just been to see him and understand there is no hope."

"Tomorrow it is my turn to celebrate Mass in his community chapel. Immediately after Mass I will go to the hospital to bring

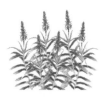

him comfort with the sacraments of the Church. Will that be all right?"

"Certainly. Please let me thank you in advance. Do you think we should start preparing his imminent funeral?"

"Only God knows when it will be..."

"Naturally. But my uncle's case is without hope. There is nothing else to be done; there's no cure for him." The blacksmith was adamant.

"I agree it is serious. However, for God nothing is impossible," I told him.

"Of course. All right. Thank you and goodbye." The blacksmith hurried off.

The next day, after celebrating Mass in the Navigators' Chapel, I went to the hospital. The ill man's wife, Gemma, looking stressed and worried over the serious illness of her husband, took my arm at the door:

"Father, first let me thank you for coming. Second, please tell Giovanni he has cancer. I want him to confess and be prepared for his imminent death. I am asking you this because I want my husband to go to heaven when he dies."

"Let me decide, Gemma," I told her. "Experience has taught me to treat the sick person in the most appropriate way, even in serious cases. Try to keep calm."

In the room, I found Giovanni extremely weak. Although he did not ask for information about his condition, he told me immediately in a whisper of a voice that he wished to confess, a

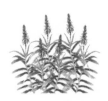

general confession, as this would be his last. He stressed that he wanted a proper job.

What an excellent state of mind, I thought with delight. It is gratifying for a priest to find the penitent person in these conditions. He does not have to motivate penitence when it already exists. There is no need to reason when the sinner already shows he has repented. Nice and easy! Just as well!

I listened to Giovanni's confession. He was repentant and, on the one hand, was aware of sin, and on the other showed limitless faith in God's mercy. I gave him absolution, the apostolic blessing, extreme unction and the viaticum. It was the best the Church has to offer in extreme cases such as Mr. Giovanni Mariani's.

I did not feel it appropriate to inform him of his extremely precarious condition as his wife had asked because, in my opinion, it was not my place; I was not the sick man's doctor. At that point, I remembered the recipe for the preparation that can cure cancer, the same recipe I had heard in the mate circle in the courtyard of the Provincialate. I went over it to refresh my memory: half a kilo of honey, two Aloe leaves and three or four tablespoons of distillate. To my mind, it seemed the same as the original recipe.

As I left the hospital, Gemma thanked me for the religious service offered to her husband. I thought I should inform her of what had happened.

"Gemma," I told her, "your husband is ready for whatever happens. He has received all one requires in such a serious case as his. With regard to your request to inform him of his illness, I did not mention it. In my opinion, it is not my place to inform him of the medical diagnosis, as I am not an expert in this field. Moreover, I know of a mixture that can cure cancer…"

"But Father, those suffering from a tumor must die! At least, that is what usually happens. I think you are trying to be kind to the family in a difficult situation like the one we are in. Thank you in any case. We are realistic which, although difficult, is necessary. Hiding the truth changes nothing."

I was wasting my breath trying to explain to Gemma that it is possible to cure cancer. She reacted the same way as other people with this problem and as I myself would react.

"With all the money spent throughout the world, how could such a simple homemade recipe perform a miracle?" She would not budge from her certainty and continued to believe her husband would die. In her mind, this dreadful fate was irremediable. When I realized I was talking to a brick wall, I decided to take action, leaving aside theories and words.

Luckily, the couple's son Rubens was on his way back from the office of the Notary, Agostino Basso, where he had been trying to put the documents concerning the estate in order. He asked me for a lift to the gate of his farm. While we were traveling, I thought to myself, "Perhaps, as I had no luck with his mother, I'll be able to convince him to try the recipe."

Throughout the journey, I tried to persuade the boy that it was in his hands to prevent his father from dying of cancer. To

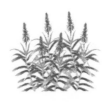

achieve this, all he had to do was apply what I would teach him. I explained and repeated it over and over.

When we reached his destination, I made him repeat the lesson. He knew it by heart. He also assured me that his sister Rejane, who was to take the place of their mother at the hospital tomorrow to give her a rest, would take the prepared blend to his father.

Satisfied at the chance of success, I said goodbye, encouraging him and imploring him to use the recipe.

I drove the rest of the way back to the parish with a clear conscience, convinced that if they followed my instructions, they could save this farmer's life.

I went back to my parish activities on my own in remote regions. Giovanni Mariani had to take second place to all the things that involved me every day. Whenever his lean figure came to mind, I hoped the drink would have the desired effect.

The week passed like all others. One morning, about eight days after giving the sick man extreme unction, I saw Rejane in front of the Municipal Building. I immediately remembered her father's disease and went up to her, anxious to find out how things were going.

"Good morning, Rejane, How are you? How's your father?"

"Good morning," she greeted me. "I'm fine, thank you. However, my father's at death's door. The doctors discharged him this morning to allow him to die at home."

"Ah, so he's at home?"

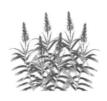

"Yes, he was discharged three days ago. There was nothing else they could do." She swallowed hard at the thought of Giovanni's death, powerless before the disease.

"Did you give him the preparation I prescribed? Did he take it correctly?"

"Yes, Father," she assured me. "It was made just as you told Rubens. I myself took it to the hospital. Father took it every day and is still taking it. But he is so weak! Excuse me for saying this, but he looks like a dead tree lying in bed. What a dreadful disease! This damned disease has ruined my father."

"Look, if he has taken the medicine, as you assure me, don't worry. All will be well. The problem is when people refuse to take it."

"You know, Father, something strange *has* happened. Did you know my father had a swelling at stomach level?"

"No, I didn't," I said.

"Yes. A swelling as large as a tennis ball. Anyway, it has disappeared!"

"Ah, then I must congratulate you, my dear, because your father is out of danger. He has won the battle against cancer. If this were not the case, then why would this swelling have gone away? On the contrary, it would be even bigger. In other words, the preparation has been successful. Hurray! Your father is all right, believe me. After a couple of weeks of convalescence, he will return to the group to work, as he has been doing for many years, for the harvest. You'll see!"

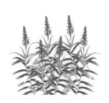

And that is what happened. Giovanni Mariani, little by little, started to eat more. After a few days, he left his bed. He started to walk up and down the room. By leaning on the wall, he managed to reach the kitchen. He then went into the yard to see his animals. Walking through the fields, he harvested the first grains of rice that became ripe. He ate the first citrus fruits of the season. He sucked the sugar cane avidly, just as he had done as a child.

Month after month, as well as taking part in the yearly harvest at the end of autumn-beginning of winter, he worked the land with oxen and plough, just as he had always done, to be ready to sow in spring.

Giovanni Mariani is still alive today at over eighty years old (he was born in 1913) in full health. He is one of the many people who managed to defeat cancer by taking the preparation being promoted in this book. Some may doubt, but the fact remains that, although he had cancer, Giovanni Mariani is alive today and is undeniable proof that the preparation can overcome this dreadful disease.

There are many men and women like Giovanni Mariani who were able to defeat cancer, each with his or her own story, which confirms the beneficial story of this first patient whose victory made me believe in the effectiveness of this system in the battle against cancer.

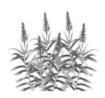

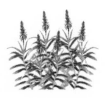

The Recipe

1. For those who have followed me to this point, it may not be necessary to repeat that I heard the recipe by word of mouth while sipping mate. It is possible that I didn't memorize it correctly, especially in view of the impact of this astounding revelation. Nonetheless, cancer can be cured!

Each time a message is transmitted by word of mouth, there is a chance that it has not been fully understood. This is perhaps the fault of the communicator or due to the limits of the receiver because of the limits of human imperfection.

In any case, I started to teach the use of the recipe I had learned, using two Aloe leaves, half a kilo (1.1 lbs.) of honey, and three spoonfuls of distillate. For many years I have taught people to use these ingredients. I was satisfied with the use of these ingredients because they had positive results similar to those described in the previous chapter. Therefore, there was no reason to change this winning recipe.

2. Later I found the same recipe to cure cancer in the book **The Pharmacy of Nature**, by Sister Maria Zatta, ed. 1988, page 14, but with significant variants. Here is the recipe, written down as found in this book:

In the early morning or after sunset pick two leaves of Aloe; wash them and remove the spines. Cut into pieces and blend them with one kilogram (2.2 lbs.) of honey and two spoonfuls of

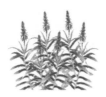

distillate. Take two spoonfuls twice a day for 10 days. Then suspend for 10 days and continue in this manner until cured.

To prevent cancer, the recipe is the same, taking only two spoonfuls a day for 10 days. In this case, the treatment is taken once a year.

The new edition of the book **The Pharmacy of Nature**, (second edition, 1993, reviewed and extended) gives the recipe on page 20, with a few modifications to the details:

In the early morning or after sunset pick two leaves of Aloe; wash them and remove the spines. Cut into pieces and blend them with one kilogram (2.2 lbs.) of honey and two spoonfuls of distillate. Take two spoonfuls twice a day for 10 days. Then suspend for 10 days and continue in this manner until cured. Do not take on an empty stomach. To prevent cancer, the recipe is the same, taking only two spoonfuls a day for 10 days. Take this treatment once a year.

3. When I organized the Pastoral Group for Health in the Parish of Santo Antonio, at Pouso Novo, Rio Grande do Sul, Mrs. Gládis Lavarda, one of the members of the group, had a stenciled print of the recipe for treating cancer. Here too there were substantial differences in the recipe, which follows. I later learned that this recipe was copied from the book **Health Through the Plants**, by Paulo Cesar de Andrade dos Santos, Ed. Mundo Jovem, pages 37-8.

The following is found under the heading *General Recipes*, at the term "cancer":

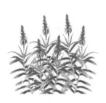

Ingredients: three large Aloe leaves, half a kilo (1.1 lbs.) of honey, a spoonful of distillate.

How to prepare: to prepare the preparation against cancer, the rules below must be strictly observed:

- the Aloe plant must be at least five years old;
- pick the leaves in the dark;
- after five days without rain;
- do not pick with frost;
- prepare in the dark;
- prepare immediately after picking;
- keep the preparation in a dark jar in the fridge;
- take in the dark (Note: the reason is that both sunlight and artificial light must be avoided because Aloe contains a substance that reacts to cancer and, in contact with either sunlight or artificial light, this automatically loses its effect);
- clean the Aloe with a dry cloth;
- cut and blend together with the honey and distillate.

How to take:

- to avoid cancer, everyone should take the preparation at least once a year, one tablespoonful three times a day, for 10 days.
- to cure cancer, take two tablespoonfuls three times a day for 10 days; stop for 10 days and then take it again for another 10 days; continue to take it until completely

cured. (**Note:** Cancer will be cured when it is in the initial phase, as the more advanced the phase, the more difficult it is to cure.)

4. In the same period, I came across the book **Saude pela Alimentacao**, (Eating for Health) by Father Adelar Primo Rigo, with other variants of the recipe. His recipe was more similar to Sister Maria Zatta's, as can be seen below:

- Honey, Aloe and distillate. In the morning or after sunset, pick two leaves of Aloe, wash them and remove the spines. Cut into pieces and blend them with one kilogram (2.2 lbs.) of honey and two tablespoonfuls of distillate. Take two tablespoonfuls twice a day for 10 days. Then suspend for 10 days and continue in this manner until cured.
- The recipe to prevent cancer is the same. Take only two tablespoonfuls for 10 days. Take this treatment once a year.

5. In October 1995 in the new Provincialate of the Friars Minor, in via Juca Batista 330, Ipanema, Porto Alegre (RS), I was able to photocopy the original recipe, the same one that I had learned of in the old Provincialate, in via Sao Luis, 64, Santana, Porto Alegre (RS). This recipe had been passed from hand to hand among the simple folk in the suburbs of Rio Grande, the sea port of Rio Grande do Sul, from the time Father Arno Reckziegel had written it down on a piece of wrapping paper. This is the oldest, chronologically speaking. As can be seen below, it too has variants.

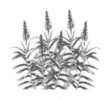

Cancer preparation:
- Two Aloe leaves, as old as possible (4-5 years), pick in the dark (morning or evening), after six days without rain;
- remove the spines, cut into pieces and blend;
- add a cup of honey;
- one spoonful of distillate;
- place in the fridge.

How to take:
- One tablespoonful three times a day (preferably before meals) for 10 consecutive days
- Stop for 10 days and then start again.

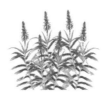

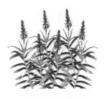

The Conclusive Recipe

Encouraged that the recipe I had learned by word of mouth had cured Giovanni Mariani and many other people over a period of at least five years, I was determined not to abandon it. I would never have replaced it with Sister Maria Zatta's recipe, although I consider this nun of the Immaculate Heart of Mary an expert in her job and a person with immense experience, a true living computer on the subject of recipes. For the same reason, I have never been able to use the recipe contained in the stenciled copy brought by Mrs. Gládis Lavarda.

In other words, I had personal experience that had worked in many cases. What information did I possess to change one recipe or use another? Until then, the one I normally used had given satisfactory results. If I were to choose another, on what information would I base my trust in, or denial of, its efficacy? Would I give in to something new? The only knowledge I had was what I had obtained first hand and that I transmitted by word of mouth.

However, I confess that I ended up changing the early recipe for practical reasons. Basically, this can be summarized in a single fact. The compound, prepared according to the recipe I had used until then, was too sweet and caused a certain degree of revulsion, especially in those with liver problems. How was I to solve this problem?

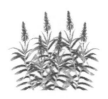

First, I compared the different recipes with each other, observing the variants. Each had substantial differences, some extremely significant. I couldn't have chosen one over another without good reason.

I put my trust in experience, the teacher of life. Only this could safely and objectively teach me what the ideal recipe was to be.

And with a view to life, my hesitancy in changing the recipe was essentially based on the erroneous information that Aloe was a toxic plant. It is clear that, if this were true, it could have been fatal to increase the dosage. Now, life is truly the greatest gift. It cannot be taken lightly, joking with it or putting it at risk without due cause, nor can people be used as guinea pigs.

Use of the recipe in daily life gave me the courage to stop using the old recipe, which I had relied on until then, as it had always given positive results.

I can assure you that this change happened by chance. The first fact that led me to make this decision was the healing of the secretary of the Terra Santa School in Bethlehem, Israel, who was suffering from cancer of the throat. I had heard that he had lost his voice several months before and could only communicate with gestures. When the principal of the school, Father Rafael Caputo, OFM, informed me of the secretary's true condition, I offered to try to help him regain his health so he could return to his duties in the school.

I prepared the mixture using the traditional recipe, two Aloe leaves, half a kilo (1.1 lb.) of honey, and distillate.

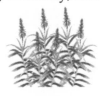

After finishing the first jar, which lasted 15 days, the sick man had medical tests before starting the second. The tests showed the preparation had stopped the disease from advancing, so the tests done before the Aloe treatment and those done after 15 days of treatment had practically the same results. Enthusiastic over the positive result (at least the disease had not spread!), his daughter Mary, the wife of a doctor, perhaps through the wish to see her father rid of the disease, prepared the next jar, using three Aloe leaves blended together with the half kilo of honey and distillate. After a pause of one week, she gave him the third dose. After about two months of treatment, the sick man started to make his first sounds, a sure sign the disease had been defeated.

To end the story of this case, the secretary went back to his job at the school. At the time this was written, he has been back at work for four years. According to Sister Veronica Mancadori from Cagliari, a teacher in this school who has known the patient for over 15 years, his voice is as good as ever.

A second episode that caused me to change the old recipe, so dear and based on experience, was the story of Shucri, driver for the Aida Franciscan Sisters of the Immaculate Heart of Mary. Having heard that people had been cured of tumors by taking the preparation I had prescribed, Shucri got up the courage to overcome his natural shyness and asked me to prepare a dose for his brother-in-law, who had an enormous open sore on his neck from cancer of the throat. Naturally I gave him the preparation, hoping he could save his relative's life.

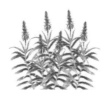

Satisfied with the result of the initial cure (the sore had healed over), Shucri wanted a second jar. This time he prepared the blend on his own. He blended four Aloe leaves with the same amount of honey and distillate as usual.

I was curious to know how he had prepared the second dose. When he told me he had used four Aloe leaves, I said: "But I told you to use two leaves."

"I know," he said.

"Why did you double the dosage?" I asked, "and what will we do if the sick man dies?"

"Don't worry, Father. He has his voice back; he can talk again. As the leaves were small and dry, I put four in the blender. However, to balance it up, I put a little more araq (Arab distillate) in!"

"Oh, well," I said, "if the sick man is better, it is clear the plant is not toxic, at least not in the quantity you used. Of course, you used too much distillate and doubled the number of leaves. Imagine that!"

It was following facts such as these and the study of the variants in the other recipes that had come to my knowledge that I made the decision to change the recipe. In my journeys, in contact with other people and cultures, I began to doubt that Aloe was toxic, as is the case with avelco, another plant used to combat cancer. I learned that the Mexicans use it as salad. In Venezuela, they swallow the gel from the Aloe at breakfast, with a few drops of honey to make it less bitter.

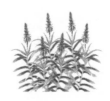

As this was the situation, it seems that the toxicity of Aloe is not such an important factor. In any case, old and wise advice continues to be the best: it is the dosage, the amount administered, that marks the limit between medicine and poison. The correct amount is always the most prudent choice. With a view to this, the reader can rest easy. We shall return to this subject in more detail, proving that Aloe is by no means toxic, as people say. If you find it useful, read the specific chapter on this subject.

After 10 years of experience in Brazil, in the East and also in Europe (especially Italy, Switzerland and Portugal), I feel I can write down the recipe without fear of erring.

---

1. Half a kilo (1.1 lbs.) of honey. Do not use synthetic or refined honeys and general fakes.

2. Between 40 and 50 ml (6-8 tsps) of grappa, whisky, cognac, etc. (pure alcohol, wine, beer and liqueurs cannot be used). **Note:** 40-50 ml is the equivalent of a measure of whisky or a small coffee cup.

3. 350 grams (.77 lbs.) of Aloe arborescens leaves. Use three or four leaves, depending on their length.

The person making up the preparation at home needn't be too meticulous. The three components must be as near as possible to the quantities above. The efficacy of the preparation will not be affected by exaggerating a bit or forgetting a detail. Therefore, there is no need for precise measurements using the scales.

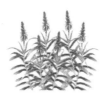

Instead, learn to prepare the blend freely, as if preparing a small corner of the garden to sow with flowers or vegetables. Use your sight and common sense. The essential thing is that these components are included in the beverage. It is the combination of the components that gives the desired effect.

Remove dust or any other impurities left on the Aloe leaves by nature. Use an old cloth, dry or dampened, or a sponge, without getting the leaves wet (no water is used in the preparation).

Use a sharp knife to remove the spines along the edge of the leaves, chopping with a light hand, in one fell swoop from the top toward the bottom. To help the work of the blender, cut the leaves into pieces, as if preparing a normal blend, and blend the three components together.

Blend well, shredding all the material. In about a minute (depending on the power of the appliance), a kind of green mixture is produced, and it's ready. You have prepared the recipe that can even cure cancer.

We have seen that the authors are not in agreement over the exact quantities of ingredients used to make the preparation and, believing that each person has gained personal experience concerning the advice offered, I advise readers to choose the best variant of this recipe – the one they prefer, sweeter or more bitter, as they all promise to heal, which is the ultimate objective. It is necessary to prepare the blend using the ingredients given, complying approximately with the amounts prescribed.

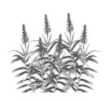

Each time someone has cancer, prepare the mix with one Aloe leaf in half a kilo (1.1 lbs.) of honey and grappa, or with two, three or even four and more leaves. The important thing is to use the recipe.

By using the recipe, you can offer the sick person the chance of being cured. You too have a role in this battle. It's up to you to decide.

Note: The day I was typing these pages, I came across the book **Health Basics – Home Remedies**, by Sister Flavia Birck, a text used in the Social Action of the Diocese of Santa Cruz do Sul, R.S. Brazil.

With regard to the recipe using Aloe to cure cancer, a variant I deemed worthy of mention is found on Page 9, namely Xarope (this is not syrup!) de Babosa:

- 2 large Aloe leaves
- ½ kilo of honey
- 2 spoonfuls of distillate

Preparation:
Remove the spines from the Aloe and cut into pieces. Add honey and blend until smooth, adding the distillate. Store in the fridge.

Dosage:
- **Prevention of cancer:** take one tablespoonful on an empty stomach before lunch and dinner.

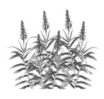

- **Cure for cancer:** take the preparation for 10 days. Stop for 10 days. Repeat the operation.

On page 19, paragraph 19, it says: Cancer: avoid it using a natural food. **Recipe:** blend two leaves (½ kilo, or 1.1 lbs.) of Aloe cut into pieces without the spines. Add ½ kilo (1.1 lbs) of honey and two tablespoons of distillate. Blend until smooth. Store in a dark jar in the fridge. **Dosage:** one tablespoonful morning and evening for 10 days. Stop for 10 days and repeat for another 10 days.

Do not waste or damage nature! If you cut a stalk of Aloe to use the leaves, plant it and you will obtain another Aloe plant – true wealth, within hand's reach.

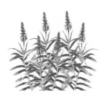

How to Take the Preparation

We have already mentioned that there is disagreement on the exact quantities of each ingredient used to prepare the compound. You may even have noticed that there are substantial differences between one variant and another. To refresh your memory, it is worthwhile mentioning that these range from two Aloe leaves in one kilo of honey to three Aloe leaves in half a kilo of honey. This is quite a difference!

We also find similar differences when the authors explain how to take the preparation (or in the quantities) both to cure cancer and to prevent the disease. So, follow me patiently:

- In her book **The Pharmacy of Nature**, Sister Maria Zatta says: Take two spoonfuls of the preparation twice a day for 10 days. This is the prescription for those suffering from cancer. In another paragraph, she describes how to prevent the disease: To prevent cancer, the recipe is the same, taking only two spoonfuls a day for 10 days. Take this treatment once a year.
- Then, Paulo Cesar de Andrade dos Santos, on page 38 of his book, **Health Through Plants**, under the heading *How to take*, says: To prevent cancer, everyone should take the preparation at least once a year, one tablespoonfuls 3 times a day, for 10 days. Instead, to cure a cancer, take two spoonfuls of the preparation 3 times a day for 10 days;

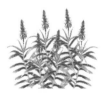

stop for 10 days and then repeat the cure for another 10 days, and so on until completely cured.

It can be seen how there are considerable variants in the written recipe of the recipe.

Just imagine how many variations can be found when the recipe is transmitted by word of mouth, from generation to generation!

I learn of these variations directly from patients, over the telephone.

- Sister Arcangela from Rome, who had cancer already in metastasis, took our preparation for 75 days without a pause, even though she had been told of the importance of stopping for at least a week after finishing the first jar. She said she acted out of desperation in the agonizing search for a way to be cured. She had heard that the Aloe preparation might be her only hope. The result is that she has fully recovered from cancer and does voluntary work at a hospital in Trastevere in the Eternal City.
- Sister Elena from the Lebanon, a Carmelite with an active life who lives and works in the port city of Haifa, Israel, modified the recipe by adding 750 grams (1.6 lbs.) of a mixture based on Aloe and distillate (araq) to 500 grams (1.1 lbs.) of honey. This overexaggeration worried me. However, I eventually calmed down after hearing that

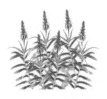

the patient who had taken these elephant-sized doses had been cured of cancer.

- Girolamo Giacomo, from Monreale in Palermo, Italy, was suffering from cancer of the liver and told he had only a few days to live. He has been taking a large spoonful of the preparation every day for the last two years. This is his way of keeping the disease under control, although he cannot defeat it even by doubling the dose (he has already tried).

Although the authors do not agree on quantities, composition of the preparation or instructions regarding the dose to take, they all agree on the three ingredients of the recipe; these are indispensable.

Along the way, we shall provide clarifications aimed at giving a scientific explanation to this recipe. Could common practice, with all its variants, find scientific backing? Or does science help make the recipe worthy of trust, or is it only a popular belief? What would the results be if these ingredients were subjected to laboratory tests?

If science could guarantee that by using these ingredients a person could be cured of or prevent cancer, we might reach a unanimous opinion on the quantities of the three components that are used to prepare the blend. This would end all discussions.

Note: After preparation of the blend, it is normal for the honey – the heaviest ingredient – to sink to the bottom of the jar;

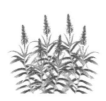

the foamy part tends to rise to the top. Shake the jar well to mix the ingredients before taking it.

If you have a tumor, during the Aloe treatment, collaborate in the battle to try to defeat the disease, to bring yourself back to health; stop eating meat and animal products. Replace these foods with fruit, vegetables and cereals.

If there are people affected by degenerative diseases (Parkinson's, Alzheimer's, or others), where Aloe does not guarantee total healing, tell the sick person to try this preparation. Strengthening the immune system will give some relief and benefits, improving the quality of life. It may be worthwhile to take this initiative: it has the advantage of having no side effects and being available inexpensively.

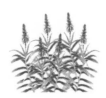

Questions and Answers

I imagine you have many questions to ask. In this chapter, I answer a series of questions people have asked me in various circumstances, over the telephone and in person, during conferences.

The recipe to cure cancer, or prevent it, may seem simple. I agree. It can be compared, as was said in the mate circle, to discovering something as plain as the nose on your face. I wish to add a few explanations to clarify the subject. I have taken the liberty of asking questions the reader might ask. Perhaps these are not exactly what you wish to know, but I believe they are pretty close. Imagine that you are asking these questions.

Q. **Why is bees' honey used to prepare the blend? Could sugar be used instead if no honey is available?**

A.   Honey is used because, since ancient times, it has been considered an excellent, genuine food with many qualities. Honey is able to move to all parts of the body – the remote corners. It is the vehicle that carries the Aloe, which cleanses and removes the impurities it finds along the way. This procedure performs general cleansing of the entire body – especially the blood – and can heal cancer and other correlated diseases, such as rheumatism, arthrosis, etc.

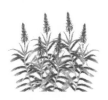

Everyone knows blood is vital to the human body. Its function is identical to the fuel in a motor vehicle. We know the engine will not work long if the fuel is poor quality.

The opposite is also true. The engine will perform better and last longer if top quality fuel is used. Purified blood is directly responsible for the health of the body and consequently for the life of the person. By taking our preparation, you invest in your health, as you are working toward improving the quality of your life. It is important to cleanse at least once a year. This is as necessary as normal maintenance. Consider yourself lucky you do not have a tumor. Take precautions against cancer and free yourself of a host of ailments by preparing your own dose of Aloe at least once a year.

Q. Why is distillate included in the ingredients?

A.   Distillate on its own may seem the least important ingredient. The first explanation I received on the importance of using distillate was that in far-off places, in caves where there is still no electricity, people don't have fridges. Without this appliance, the product could go bad. Distillate is used to preserve the preparation, preventing it from perishing. This is a plausible explanation.

Later I heard an odd although pertinent reason: the distillate is used to dilate the blood vessels. To clarify this, I was given an explanation of this function with reference to clinical cases. When a patient has circulation problems, he is prescribed a dose of whisky to try to correct this deficiency. This explanation seems logical and the example has provided me with a better understanding of the function of the distillate. It also became clear that, in older people especially, dilated blood vessels would speed up the cleansing action of the Aloe and honey.

Later I learned the true function of the distillate from scientific research. The third component of the preparation is not used by chance or whim. The explanation is that when the Aloe leaf is cut, it gives off a viscous, stringy, bitter, greenish liquid rich in properties called aloin. The human body is unable to absorb this fully if it is not dissolved in the distillate.

I wish to stress that the first two explanations are not without sense. The first makes us understand that the blend can also be kept out of the fridge without going bad, in the cupboard or dresser, as long as it is away from light. The second points out the vasodilator function of the distillate.

With regard to distilled drinks, it must be mentioned that the following are all equally effective: Brazilian grappa (cachaça), cognac or whisky, Mexican tequila, Italian grappa, Dutch bols, araq from Palestine and other Arab countries, and others. Neither wine nor beer must be used, as they are fermented, with lower concentrations of alcohol. If necessary, they have to be used in greater quantities. No kinds of liqueur must be used, as these are sugar-based products.

Q. What is Aloe?

A. Throughout the world, it is known as Aloe, with the variant aloes, a plant full of medicinal sap, from the Liliaceous genus (Aloe succotrina, Aloe humilis, Aloe perfoliata, Aloe vulgaris, Aloe arborescens, Aloe vera or barbadensis, Aloe ferox, etc.), similar to pineapple, but smaller. Its leaves are thick and serrated. As soon as it is touched by a sharp object, it releases a viscous liquid (similar to slavers – baba in Portuguese – from the mouth of the ox when it chews corn, cassava root or a hard object). This is why Brazilians call Aloe Babosa (the drooler), with a strong characteristic smell, a greenish color, viscous and very bitter.

In Spanish-speaking countries, the plant is known as saliva, with countless variants.

The term "Aloe" comes from Arabic. It passed from Arabic through Greek and Latin to reach us, to give a scientific name to the plant. Its original meaning was bitter and glossy or transparent because, when the skin is removed, the gel released is similar to a block of washed ice.

The leaves of this plant can vary in size from twenty to sixty centimeters, (8-24 inches) according to the quality of the soil, the amount of water present, and its exposure to sunlight. There is a shoot in the center of the plant, the end of which is covered in white, yellow, orange or red flowers, depending on which variety it is. The flowers appear at the end of autumn-beginning of winter and last until the end of the season. The most common Aloe (arborescens) has an orange flower.

When the large succulent leaves are fully grown, they are ready for our preparation. If we were to lift the green skin of a leaf slightly (the outer part), we would see the pulpy, flexible, limp part, similar in color to an ice cube that has been washed, or glossy and transparent like a piece of wet glass.

Are you tired of this lengthy description? The objective is to make the plant easier to identify. If you turn to nature to prepare a tisane, it is essential to know how to identify the plants.

There are hundreds, perhaps thousands of different types of Aloe. Are they all useful? Are they all efficacious to the same extent? Are some more or less so? Do they all contain the active ingredient against cancer?

With these questions to answer, I went to the Botanical Gardens of Palermo in Sicily, Italy, where I set a challenge for the director, Francesco Maria Raimondo, asking him to examine the 140 different types of Aloe found there, with the help of a botanist. He said he would. I have been trying to find the solution to the case for a long time. The answer would simplify everything. Imagine if all types of Aloe were just as effective! There would be no margin for error.

Until we have data and valid experiences to confirm this, I will continue to use the type of Aloe that is used as a hair tonic, which I have vast experience of. This type of Aloe has always given good results. Are there other more potent varieties of this plant? Are there types that are more toxic, and to what extent? It is an unexplored field still to be investigated.

Note: Garlic and onion, which we use every day in the kitchen, also belong to the lilaceum family.

Q.   Why take the preparation before meals?

A.   Before meals, pepsin – the enzyme of gastric acid capable of hydrolyzing proteins – that aids digestion, is ready to start work. When the stomach is empty, all the passages are empty. This facilitates the work of the preparation and makes it possible to transport it anywhere in the body. Therefore, it is fundamental to take it before meals, when pepsin is ready to start work.

However, if the preparation is taken after meals, pepsin is tired from the work performed during digestion. At this point, it gives in or requests a well earned rest. If the preparation is taken after meals, it might not be as effective.

Q.   Why do Sister Maria Zatta and other authors recommend picking the Aloe leaves in the morning, before sunrise, or in the evening after sunset?

A. Because when there is no sun, there are no ultraviolet and infrared rays to damage the plant. This wise advice by Sister Maria Zatta is a prudent measure. It should be followed with all medicinal plants and herbs picked for this purpose. Specifically, Aloe must not be picked in sunlight as the substance in it that reacts to cancer could, if exposed to light, lose its effectiveness as an active ingredient to combat the tumor.

Q. **Should one avoid picking the Aloe leaves immediately after it has rained?**

A. Yes, Aloe leave are porous, so they absorb rain. This preparation does not require a lot of water, as the plant itself is 95% water. The leaves should be picked one week after the last rainfall.

    Avoid using leaves exposed to pollution – near motorways, sewers, or in closed, smoky environments. Because of their porosity, Aloe leaves that have absorbed toxic substances are totally unsuitable to make the preparation.

Q. **What age should the Aloe plant be to be considered suitable to provide the leaves required?**

A. A five-year-old plant is ideal. If necessary, younger plants may be used. There will be cases where you will have to make do with 95% compliance. However, as far as possible, you should try to stick to the indications given.

Q. **Is the person with cancer always cured after taking the preparation with its three ingredients, using the recipe given previously?**

A. When someone who has cancer, proven by medical diagnosis, makes use of this preparation, there are three hypothetical situations:

1) The person is totally cured, notwithstanding the type of cancer or how far it has spread. Even a terminally ill person can be cured. We have a great deal of information that confirms this, though it may seem miraculous. When you understand the full potential of Aloe, you will understand that it is not a miracle in the true sense of the word, but something found in nature, created by God. We shall deal with this subject in a separate chapter. Be patient.

2) Medical tests show the disease has been halted. In other words, the disease has not spread. Without the use of Aloe, the cancer would inevitably have continued to spread. However, in this case, the results of tests are more or less the same as before, with only insignificant variations in either direction. Without this cure, the disease would have spread considerably.

3) The cure has had no effect and, according to medical tests, the disease continues to spread unrestrained. **Note:** I have had experience with all three situations.

Q. **Can you go into the three situations in more depth? What should one do, especially in situations 2) and 3), when the objective of healing the patient has not been attained?**

A. That's a good question! Let's comment on the three situations adequately.

Situation 1) If you are in this condition, that's wonderful! Congratulations! The product has produced the results hoped for. The person has been cured. There is no harm in preparing a second jar as a preventive to guarantee and strengthen the cure. In any case, wait a few months, repeat the dose and be optimistic. It is advisable to repeat the cure within one year.

Situation 2) You have obtained a great result. You are on the right track; just persevere. In mathematical terms, you have reached 50% of the overall result. With another dose, you will reach your goal: total healing. It is essential to repeat the treatment without fear. You must repeat it as often as required to obtain complete healing.

Do not stop halfway through the work; if you do, all will be lost. The cancer that seems to have been defeated will double its strength and attack with greater vehemence.

If you do not repeat the cure, before long you will be dead. If you do not take the treatment, this is inevitable. Cancer is like a sick person. During the illness, it is not interested in anything. However, during convalescence, after the illness has been defeated, the appetite returns to regain lost strength. Try to imagine the voracity with which the cancer will devour your body after having lost ground during the Aloe cure. It will try to regain it. In a short time, it will consume its master. A typical example of this is the case of Sister Margherita, who had breast cancer. After taking one jar of the preparation in the Italian Hospital in Haifa (Israel), she felt much better and went back to her work without undergoing the routine tests and examinations by a specialist. Less than one year later, she was dead. Her case notes are important proof that stopping advance of the disease is an excellent result, but not enough. It is essential to repeat the dose and remain in the care of competent doctors.

Situation 3) You had no result with the treatment. Don't despair. You know you are living with the Beast. You must tame it. And you will manage. You have the weapons. Use them fearlessly and with faith. This is your only chance to defeat it, but it is a concrete and true opportunity. Take another jar of the preparation. Even if your case is extremely serious, even in the terminal phase, it doesn't matter. Do not get upset and let what other people are saying distract you. Where there's life, there's hope. Therefore, you must fight for your life, the most precious gift you possess. When you finish the jar, wait one week and start another. If need be, repeat the dose twice, three times, four times. Just do it. Persevere. Persist to free yourself of the disease. Do not give in to the disease; you are stronger than the Beast. Your personal endeavor and your will to live have a valid ally in Aloe!

Allow me to give you some important advice: if, after having taken four jars of the preparation, you still have not achieved the objective and been cured, take a double dose. Instead of one tablespoonful before breakfast, lunch and dinner, take two spoonfuls each time until you are cured. This advice is backed by the vast experience of those who agree with me and support me.

Q. **I know I have cancer, because tests confirm it and my doctor has diagnosed it. I have taken the Aloe remedy and feel much, much better. How will I know whether I am completely cured?**

A. This is extremely simple. Just repeat the medical tests. Compare the new results with the previous ones and you will be able to clarify your ideas and find the peace of mind you need. Only this system will give definite results. It is very important to compare the test results, first to check your situation and protect you and second, the results will show whether you need another jarful.

Ideally, you should know your medical situation before starting the Aloe treatment. If tests show you have a malignant tumor, start taking Aloe. When you have finished, repeat the tests meticulously. Compare them to the former ones. After this, you will find yourself in one of the three situations above. You will know what measures to take. Keep calm, even if you find yourself in situation 3). If this is the case, you already know what to do: in situations 2) and 3), take another jar of the product. And persist. You will manage to obtain your objective, I assure you.

Q.   I thank God that I am in perfect health and do not think I have cancer. However, as this disease is extremely common, I would like to take precautions against it. How should I act? What must I do?

A.   Prepare the compound with the same ingredients and take it in the same doses as a person with cancer. As you know you don't have cancer, there is no need to repeat the dose, as in the case of a sick person. By taking this remedy once a year, you will be sure to keep cancer at bay. By taking the recipe at least once a year, your body will be healthy and your blood purified. And one does not get cancer in these conditions, believe me!

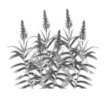

Q.   What exactly is cancer?

A.   Cancer has always existed, though it is much more
frequent today, I would even say to an alarming degree. It
has become part of the routine of modern man. The disease
destroys the body cells, and if not defeated in time, it
weakens the cells ruthlessly through the impurities deposited
in it. The toxic cells, lacking in some substances and
overloaded with others, in turn become ill and collapse
and start to attack the healthy cells. In time, this fight
exhausts the body because of the prevalence of the
diseased cells. There may be no pain initially, but a tumor
slowly forms. This frees toxic substances and attacks
healthy cells with tremendous violence until the body can
no longer withstand the fight. At that point, the cancer
becomes fatal. This disease has countless variants that
affect all parts of the body, internally and externally.

Cancer is proof of the body's incredible intelligence and
capacity to adapt and defend itself. It could be compared
to a cleaning operation performed in an environment, a
house or room. After sweeping the floor, the dirt is
collected and thrown away. Everything is thrown into bins
used to prevent pollution. In this way, the body frees itself
of internal surplus and attempts to rid itself of damaging
substances. This is when a tumor is triggered in a certain
part of the body. It is like a volcano. The heat underground
eventually erupts. In the same way, the body shrewdly

collects toxins and accumulates them in a certain organ in an attempt to save the rest of the body.

Regarding degenerative diseases such as AIDS, cancer, scleroses, dystrophies, etc., orthodox medicine continues to impose and propose aggressive treatment as a remedy (operate = cut) each time the disease is localized. It then attempts to close the wound with radiotherapy, chemotherapy and similar applications, as if by extracting the sick organ, the patient will be healed. Normally what happens is that once the center of infection has been removed, the patient's inevitable journey toward death continues. No healing takes place, the cancer attacks some other part of the body, and the sick person enters the stage of metastasis. The end is imminent.

This recipe heals the sick body through purification. It fortifies the immune system, weakened through the years by some form of physical, psychic or spiritual conflict. In the chapter on the properties of Aloe, we will see how it helps the weakened body.

Q.   What are the causes of cancer?

A. 1: Cancer originates from variations in physical condition. Man lives in an increasingly polluted environment. Pollution occurs in the increasing decline in the quality of food, drink and air. We can mention Chernobyl,

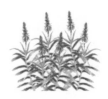

atomic explosions, the hole in the ozone layer, pesticides, preservatives, motor vehicles, and so on.

2: Cancer is caused by *psychic pollution*. Great emotional shock, such as kidnapping of an only child, lack of incentive to live, the unfaithfulness of a partner, for adolescents the separation of their parents, the loss of a dear friend, the failure of a project related to life or business, overwork, constant worry, the loss of a great love, etc.

3: Cancer can be caused by *spiritual pollution* and a bad conscience. It is easy to state, "One sin more or one sin less makes no difference!" Of course it makes a difference! How can a person who has had an abortion or killed his or her child have a clear conscience? Hate, envy, anger, and a thirst for revenge eat away at the human being. We learn that the human body is formed of soul and body (Council of Trent); today it is reasonable to add a third element, the spirit. These three elements are present in a single being (in the same manner as Father, Son and Holy Ghost, three distinct individuals, forming one God).

We know if one element enters into conflict or suffers damage, the others suffer the consequences, just as in different circumstances they would reap any benefits. The three elements are connected. People get sick because they are *polluted physically, psychically or spiritually*. To heal them, it is necessary to reactivate their immune system, which is so weak it risks collapse. My recipe can perform this recovery.

My recipe performs a cleansing operation. It wrings out the sponge that has absorbed so many toxins in the attempt to act as a safety valve. Without any surgical operation, the cleansing operation of the entire body is performed naturally.

Q.   What symptoms does a person with cancer have? Can this type of disease be predicted?

A.   This question is answered by a specialist, Dr. Mario Henrique Osanai, oncologist and surgeon at Santa Rita Hospital, Santa Casa Hospital Complex in Porto Alegre: "There are changes in the person's physical conditions which do not necessarily prove the presence of a tumor. However, it is necessary to consult a specialist who will investigate the causes of these changes meticulously. The main symptoms are wounds that do not heal, swellings in any part of the body, lumps or hardened parts, changes in color, variations in size, blood loss, itching or pain in specific points (moles, wounds or rashes), fragile or broken teeth, difficulty in urinating or swallowing, or loss of weight without any apparent cause. Blood loss from the mouth, nose and vagina (after sexual intercourse or after menopause), blood in the urine, feces or catarrh, change in voice (permanent hoarseness)." See *Vivere Meglio* in the publication **Hora Zero**, of Porto Alegre, January 11, 1996. If you have any of these symptoms, consult your doctor. And use a jar of Aloe as a preventive cure and all will be well.

Q. What types of cancer can be cured by this preparation?

A. As the preparation cleanses the body totally, it is easy to understand that this treatment can truly cure any type of cancer. It may seem that I am exaggerating, but this is not the case.

If you find this impossible, try to reason with me. If cancer is caused by all the different impurities we allow to enter our bodies, it is evident that the cleansing performed by Aloe will renew the blood, strengthen the weakened immune system and automatically restore us to health.

We have news of healings that have taken place all over the world, throughout the five continents, with patients who had cancer of the:

Brain	Cerebellum	Lungs	Liver	Prostate
Uterus	Ovaries	Tubes	Breast	Throat
Bone	Skin	Intestine	Rectum	Bladder
Kidneys	Lymphatic system		Blood system	
Spinal column				

I could provide names, addresses and phone numbers of people who have been cured with my simple, inexpensive, innocent recipe. But this is ethically unacceptable. There are people who do not accept the fact that they have had cancer. Some even avoid pronouncing the word cancer, calling it a serious illness, serious as it inevitably leads its victims to their grave. This sensibility must be respected.

Q.   In your opinion, can cancer be transmitted? In other words, can the disease be caught?

A.   Scholars do not agree on this point. Until this matter has been clarified, the question will remain open from a scientific viewpoint.

The subject can only be dealt with here out of curiosity. Therefore, I offer an explanation that I deem most logical. According to me, cancer cannot be transmitted. On what grounds do I base this conclusion? One only has to reason.

By keeping the blood and body in good condition, it is not possible to become contaminated. It is obvious that incorrect eating habits and abuse can make us more liable to get the disease, as children tend to copy both the good and bad habits of their parents. How can cancer or any other disease nourish itself in a healthy body that is purified regularly? Therefore, the secret lies in keeping the body constantly clean.

Don't worry if you have to visit a person with cancer. You will not catch the disease. If cancer were contagious, every doctor, nurse and employee in a cancer hospital would have it. Have faith. Cancer cannot be transmitted, above all to a healthy body.

Q. If someone with cancer is having radiotherapy, chemotherapy or other treatment, intends having surgery or is taking medicines prescribed by the doctor, are there any contraindications to taking the Aloe, honey and distillate preparation?

A. If the person is having traditional treatment or taking medicines prescribed by his doctor, he can use this preparation as well. Actually, I have heard of patients who, by taking the dose of Aloe before having chemotherapy, were able to overcome the unpleasant side effects better: loss of hair (and even teeth at times), fever, vomiting, diarrhea, nausea. Some people did not even lose their hair. Others had only a little nausea for a few hours, but with no fever. Others stopped using cortisone and morphine after just one week of taking the Aloe treatment. If someone is taking homeopathic treatment, this does not need to be suspended as the Aloe treatment can be added.

For a question of personal coherence and respect for the opinions of others, I never advise sick people to give up orthodox treatment in favor of our method. I have great reverence for the person's freedom of choice and believe freedom to be man's greatest gift. You must use it as you

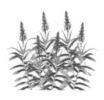

deem fit, following your conscience, for your own good and for the good of your health.

It is worthwhile repeating here that the treatment proposed is simple, natural and inexpensive. Anyone can use it and may solve their problem. If the treatment is successful, people can go back to their normal lives, totally cured, without being disfigured, even in the case of cancer in the terminal phase. Medical tests will provide the proof of complete healing.

Why don't science and medicine, with their enormous capacities in research, open the doors to more honest experiences so that humanity can beat the serious problem of cancer? Perhaps science does not wish to find the solution to this problem. Perhaps it is better for the solution to remain hidden to safeguard much greater interests. If this is the case, then this is a Mafia, and the Mafia must be exposed for man to free himself of its diabolic anger.

I am not challenging anyone. On the contrary, my proposal is that all forces should unite to solve the problem once and for all. This is not just a job for medicine, which must work side by side with other scientific disciplines, to work from an interdisciplinary viewpoint that considers the human being as a whole.

Any contribution, even the most simple, must be taken into consideration when the overall good of mankind is at stake.

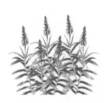

Q. **In your experience, have there been cases of people with cancer who have died after taking the treatment proposed in this book? How can a person die of this disease if they have taken the proposed treatment, which is considered to be efficacious?**

A. There have been cases of people who have taken my treatment and died of cancer. I can give various plausible explanations for this.

1. The ingredients were not well chosen. For example, synthetic honey purchased in any old shop was used in place of genuine honey.
2. The plant was not well chosen.
3. Yellowish, almost dry leaves were used.
4. The leaves used were too young.
5. The preparation was not taken in the doses indicated.
6. After having taken the first jar regularly, in the cases of incomplete cure or no cure, the treatment was suspended and the person did not have the control tests.
7. The person became discouraged and suspended the treatment after a few days, convinced that this was just another syrup, like many others, and that it had no effect.
8. The jar lay forgotten in the fridge.
9. The preparation was taken only sporadically, when the person remembered.

10. Some unknown cause.

Q. **Why must the spines be removed from the upper part of the leaf before this is blended with the honey and distillate?**

A. The blender might not blend the spines well. If a spine were swallowed together with the preparation, it might damage the mouth, throat or stomach. Removing the spines is a precaution to prevent this. There is no other reason. If I knew of a food processor that was more powerful than the blender, I would also blend the spines, as they also have healing properties.

Remove the spines lighthandedly, without removing too much of the leaf. Just scrape or cut lightly, moving the knife downward, chopping cleanly.

Q. **Is this honey, Aloe and distillate preparation solely responsible for curing cancer and other diseases directly? How important are prayer, faith and the personal qualities of the person preparing the mixture?**

A. I believe that faith and prayer alone can heal any disease, as Jesus told us faith as small as a mustard seed, which is the smallest of all seeds, can move mountains. It is not our intention to say that prayer of any kind by someone of any

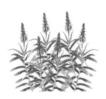

religion is of no value. Of course it is of great value. Any prayer said with faith is effective.

However, the ingredients above, created by God and taken from Mother Nature, have curative characteristics that perform miracles for anyone who takes them. If the cure is accompanied by prayer and the patient's will to be cured and spirit of cooperation, all this will undoubtedly be a great help at a psychological level. The contrary is also true, and not only when treating cancer. In any disease, the cooperation and help of the patient is fundamental for the cure. The day will come when laboratory tests prove that the preparation is solely responsible for the miracle, and not a benediction or positive force possessed by the person preparing it. The success of this treatment has nothing to do with invocations or witchcraft used by healers, nothing to do with prayer, holy water, Fatima, Lourdes, the Virgin, Guadalupe, etc.

However, we do not wish to merely say pretty words. Readers should be patient and calmly follow what has become public domain on the curative properties of this wonder of nature, Aloe. This will be discussed in a separate chapter. Those who are interested can read it; otherwise, you can go on to the next chapter. This chapter is aimed at satisfying these curiosities.

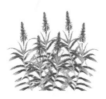

Q. Why must the leaves be cleaned before use?

A. Being exposed to weather, the plant collects dust and other dirt. Just clean the surface of the leaves with a dry or damp cloth or a sponge. The leaves must not be washed, as no water is used in the preparation. No water should be allowed to penetrate the leaves. The less water on the leaf, the better. It has already been said that it is advisable to pick Aloe for curative use one week after the last rainfall. For this reason, the advice to remove dust with a damp cloth or sponge, without water, is repeated.

Q. Are there any strange effects or problems of any type in the body of the person who has taken or is taking the Aloe treatment?

A. If there is anything causing problems to the body, this foreign substance must be expelled one way or another. Nature is wise: it can react in the most extraordinary and unimaginable ways. I have heard of people who took the preparation and had the following reactions:

1. No change or reaction.
2A. On the skin, through the pores:
    a) itching all over the body;
    b) spots, boils, tumors;
    c) eruption of a rash, like chicken pox;

      d) blisters, even on the palm of the hand or sole of the foot.
2B. Through the feces:
      a) intestinal problems, diarrhea;
      b) feces with stronger smell than normal;
      c) Malodorous flatulence (gas).
2C. Through the urine:
      a) more frequent urination;
      b) darker, almost brown, urine;
      c) urine that looks like blood mixed with water.
3. Other phenomena:
      a) vomiting;
      b) at times an attack of vomit with pus and rotten blood;
      c) aperture of three orifices under the chin in people with cancer of the throat, from which a large amount of purulent matter flows;
      d) pus oozing from the fingers or toes, or only from the big toe, which heals alone without any medication;
      e) general pain, not always localized, especially in the stomach.

I wish to stress that these ailments or disturbances only last one, two, three or a maximum of four days and are always followed by a feeling of well being and good state of mind toward everything, as is the case when convalescing. The attitude with which these problems are faced is important: the treatment must not be suspended. You must be convinced that you are on the right road, and that the toxins have found a safety valve and have left your body. You are on the way to recovery. All you have to do now is persist. If you stop taking the treatment now, all will be lost. Particularly with cancer, you already know the most appropriate way to act, as this has been discussed in depth on the previous pages.

Q.   Is it possible to list the positive effects during the cure?

A.   Let us move on from cases that have been cured of cancer, as we have already discussed this subject in depth, to talk of the healing that has taken place in people who have used the preparation as a preventive measure, as they were sure they did not have cancer. The composition of the elements and the quantities are exactly the same as those used to treat someone with cancer.

The doses are also the same. The treatment has cured or solved problems of the following nature:
- Acidity of the stomach
- Gastritis
- Ulcer
- Conjunctivitis
- Rubefaction (redness)
- Callosities (calluses)
- Spots on the skin

- Small wounds on the scalp
- Dandruff
- Rheumatism
- Arthritis
- Intestinal polyps
- Uterine polyps
- Paralysis
- Deafness
- Parkinson's Disease
- Baldness
- Sinusitis
- Lupus
- Herpes on the vaginal labia or glans
- Psoriasis
- Epilepsy
- Athlete's foot

It has also:
- Regulated bowel, eliminating constipation
- Eliminated fungal infections
- Normalized cholesterol
- Regulated blood pressure
- Stimulated the appetite
- Created thinner and softer hair
- Regulated the menstrual cycle in women who have had irregular cycles since adolescence

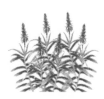

- Solved problems of night-time sweating, both in winter or summer
- Improved sexual performance in men in their forties
- Improved breathing capacity in asthma sufferers
- Regenerated an atrophied nail that was nothing but cartilage; strengthened the nail
- Prevented surgery in cases of prostate cancer in men about to be operated on
- Prevented surgery in cases of cancer of the bladder
- Eliminated persistent acne
- Eliminated catarrh, aiding expectoration
- Solved problems of bad digestion
- Improved bad breath
- Cured varicose ulcers
- Cured ulcers of the retina
- After four jars, cured from toxoplasmosis (cat virus) of the eye
- Led to recovery of sense of smell in people who had been without for many years

Q. What are the curative effects of Aloe used on its own, as a plant?

A. All the healings listed below have been confirmed by experience:
- Fungal infections
- Athlete's foot

- Callosities in 24 hours without pain
- Fistula on the gums, in the form of a deep and narrow channel
- Tumor between the toes
- Abscesses
- Dandruff, strengthening the scalp; it is a hair tonic
- Insect bites (bee, wasp, spider, mosquito, etc.)
- Scalding in domestic accidents
- Burns from x-rays
- Small cuts caused by domestic accidents (powerful cicatrisation, or healing of the wound)
- Anti-tetanus
- Eczema
- Erysipelas (acute disease of the skin and subcutaneous tissue caused by a species of hemolytic streptococcus and marked by localized inflammation and fever; also called Saint Anthony's fire)
- Ophthalmia (inflammation of the eye)
- As a suppository, it has cured hemorrhoids
- Dissolved in water, used to clear the liver
- Purifies air in a smoke-polluted room
- Works well against anemia
- Constipation: it regulates the bowel
- Rheumatism
- Cicatrizes (heals) ulcers of the retina or any other wound to the eye
- Eliminates verrucas (warts)

- Effective in combating acne
- Effective in combating worms
- Dissolved in water, it cures acidity of the stomach, gastritis, peptic ulcer

In all experiences or the majority of cases quoted, Aloe is applied locally, used externally. You can either use the gel-like substance inside the leaf, or it can be blended and the particles filtered to remove skin and spines. It must be applied with a syringe, a dropper, or cotton wool or gauze soaked in the preparation to the part with the problem.

If you think the answer to the last two questions exaggerates, you should take the time to read the list of diseases that have been overcome in the United States, on pages 40-41 of the book **Silent Healer (A Modern Study on Aloe Vera)** by Bill C. Coats, R. Ph, with Robert Ahola: In her studies and accurate reports on Aloe vera, author Carol Miller Kent gives a long list of all diseases cured with Aloe vera or barbadensis. Here it is:

- A wide range of skin diseases, including sunburn and burns from x-rays
- Ulcers
- Pustules, exanthema (a skin eruption), itchiness, abrasions, wasp, bee and mosquito stings
- Poisonous plants
- Allergic reactions
- Eruptions and reddening of the skin in children
- Chapped skin and lips

- Dandruff
- Eczema
- Dermatitis
- Impetigo (a contagious bacterial skin infection, usually of children, that is characterized by the eruption of superficial pustules and the formation of thick yellow crusts, commonly on the face)
- Psoriasis
- Urticaria (hives)
- Body wounds
- Reddening of the skin caused by heat
- Skin cancer
- Herpes zoster
- Cracks on nipples of breast-feeding mothers
- Ingrown toe nails
- Acne, brown or white marks on the skin (liver marks or chloasmata, congenital marks)
- Fibrosis, cuts, contusions, lacerations, dry or weeping lesions
- Chronic ulcers
- Abscesses
- Herpes simplex (of the mouth and lips), mouth and throat irritations
- Gingivitis
- Tonsillitis
- Staphylococcus infections
- Conjunctivitis

- Sties
- Ulcer of the cornea
- Catarrh, perforated eardrum
- Mycosis
- Fungi in general
- Itchy anus and vulva
- Vaginal infections
- Venereal wounds
- Muscle cramps
- Distortions
- Tumors
- Bursitis
- Tendonitis
- Hair loss

Used internally, it is said that Aloe vera calms headaches, insomnia, breathlessness, stomach disorders, indigestion, acidity, gastritis, peptic and duodenal ulcers, colitis, hemorrhoids, urinary infections, prostatitis (inflammation of prostate gland), inflamed fistulas and cysts, diabetes, hypertension, rheumatism and arthritis, threadworm and other parasites, cures infertility caused by amenorrhea and optimizes any imbalance caused or worsened by taking too many sugary and acidy substances.

A quick glance at the list brings to mind other diseases, including ventricular ulcer, diverticulitis, pulmonary sediments, sinusitis, moniliasis, trachoma, scleroderma, proteus infections, and snake bites. We can add that Aloe vera is a perfect deodorant, an excellent after-shave lotion, cleans metals, preserves leather paint and, to top it all, is a delicious liqueur.

I copied this long list by the American author carefully because, in Brazil, a researcher is never considered to have done anything important. All that is important must necessarily come from abroad, from the Americans, Japanese or Germans. In other words, no one is considered a prophet in his own land. And the list by the American author confirms all the results obtained by us, with the help of Aloe.

Q. How did you gain all this experience?

A. Can I tell you? I hope you won't be bored. If you're not interested, skip this part.

First, I wish to explain what I mean by experience. Experience is merely the stock of knowledge gained by helping sick people. This experience comes from careful and lengthy observation, with none of the opportunistic approach of using the sick person as a guinea pig in order to learn more. I only wished to be of help.

When I was appointed as the parish priest of Pouso Novo, a small parish on the outskirts, between Lajeado and Soledade, Rio Grande do Sul, I learned through need. This is a small, slightly developed town that the Rivers Fao and

Forqueta flow through to the right and left, the waters of which flow towards the River Taquari. Along the banks of the rivers, in the most uneven parts, there are stretches of land the people call government land, without ownership certificates or other deeds. These are places to which poor families flock, outcast from other towns, each with their own stories, mostly victims of the ambitions of the wealthy.

The sense of misfortune, lack of culture, despondency, laziness – all correlated – are indicators of general degradation: underfeeding, lack of hygiene, and lack of schooling. Illiteracy is a plague that has been transmitted from father to son through the generations since Brazil was discovered, when a host of men and women who were the scum of society were taken there from Portugal, without the colonizers ever giving a thought to the future of the colony, but wanting only to exploit it as far as possible. Only after gaining its independence did Brazil open its first university. This situation has resulted in hosts of children with lice, worms and other parasites who have been exposed to diseases and epidemics of all kinds.

After having observed this embarrassing situation, with no hope for change within traditional parameters, for six months I took the initiative to help these people excluded by society – they are God's children too! – not only by celebrating Mass when visiting the chapel or school, to then leave them to their destiny, but by promoting, alongside treatment of the spirit that seeks eternal life and all the other personal values of humankind as an inhabitant of this planet.

Unable to do the work alone, I requested the help of other well-meaning people who were sensitive to these problems but had, in the face of their complexity, acknowledged they were helpless. We should join forces urgently: the union of vital energies, each giving what they could, would undoubtedly contribute to defeating evil.

With a project scribbled down on a piece of paper placed in a waistcoat pocket, I convened those in charge of the various sectors: Parish, Secretary of the Department of Education and Culture, Secretary of Labor and Social Action, Brazilian Assistance Legion, EMATER Council (Office of Agricultural Technical Assistance), all of which cooperated, with the exception of BAL.

After having explained the project and before it was put into practice, everyone was given a photocopy and given enough time to examine and judge it.

After discussion at a second meeting, the proposal was approved with amendments. Each person who had agreed to join the work group had a task linked to his or her specific sector. This was a group performing charity work, without expecting any type of material payment, with the sole aim of promoting human beings, to try to integrate them into the community.

Instead of asking the people to come to the head-quarters, we decided to go to them, as their social conditions caused them to be extremely withdrawn. There we held conferences. All the communities, needy to a greater or lesser extent, were involved in the project, without hurting the feelings of those less advanced. The response exceeded all expectations.

In the first visits to the communities, the following subjects were covered:

1. God creates man for happiness. God does not wish man to suffer; on the contrary, it is man who looks for the road to suffering, lives together with this, either through ignorance or illusion. In most cases, the instruments to eliminate or alleviate this suffering are available. We illustrated these claims with passages from the Bible. It was the very son of God, Jesus Christ, who undertook to alleviate the suffering of man during his brief time in this world. Presentation by the Parish Priest. Duration: 10-15 minutes (the same time for the other subjects).

2. Health is a gift in the general sense. We must preserve it and look after it. We usually damage it by eating and drinking the wrong things. What should a well-balanced diet include? Which and how many vitamins and proteins does the human body require to live well and where are they found? Paper by Analice Passaia and Sandra Ines Gheno. They stressed the importance of the vegetable garden and its practical nature. They transformed the courtyard and area surrounding the school into a nursery and the secretary's office into a seed distributor,

where each pupil could collect seeds to grow in the family vegetable garden. Extremely simple. The pupils were enthusiastic about this new subject at school and told their families about the value of food, how dishes and tastes can be varied. As a result, there was a decrease in the amount of various types of meat used, which is expensive, and preference was given to the use of vegetables and grains, which are less expensive and have greater nutritional value.

Result: after the first six months of the experiment, the children had a healthier color, more energy and their performance at school had improved.

3. Along with good eating habits, hygiene is essential to guarantee good health. The first factor is water. Regular and constant cleaning of wells or tanks, which must be at a height, above the stable, far from toilets and the house, kept separate by improving the structures if necessary. Using animal excrement as fertilizer. By following these basic rules, which diseases can occur? This paper, supported by illustrative didactic material, was presented by Maria Muttoni.

4. Pesticides are also a health hazard. Purchase, storage, correct use, and elimination of packaging by the EMATER group: Jorge Lavarda, his wife Gládis and Carlos Bianchini.

Going back to what we said above, after the first cycle of conferences and checking the work performed, the group was satisfied with the results. The unanimous conclusion was that the work started must not be interrupted. The group still had a lot to offer and people still needed a great deal.

At home, the participants exchanged ideas to choose the second cycle: Diseases and treatment recipes. The same members of the group were willing to continue the work traveling to the communities, as the people wouldn't have come all the way to the center for the conferences.

The group used a procedure that led to an exchange of knowledge between the relators and those attending: among the audience were people who knew herbs and plants for tisanes (herbal teas), their purposes and doses. The objective was to encourage even the most timid to talk in public. Back at headquarters, the group consulted the existing bibliography, and confirmed whether the recipe had scientific grounding, as had been asserted during the meeting. If this was true, it became part of the group's collection of recipes. This second stage was productive for all those participating in the group.

During this second cycle, with diseases and treatment recipes, we listed a series of diseases such as cancer, acidity, gastritis, ulcer, rheumatism, etc., and the methods to combat them, as well as the battle against lice and worms that were rife among the most neglected families. The medicines to combat these diseases were sought

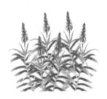

exclusively in herbs and plants that grew in abundance in the region.

The reason is that the people are extremely poor and doctors' visits are very expensive, almost prohibitive for the pockets of these people (sic!), and they cannot afford pharmaceutical medicines. After a short time, we were able to reduce doctors' visits by 90% using herbs and plants, finding domestic solutions for the symptoms of the most common diseases. From the famous aspirin (look out for its side effects), medicines were manufactured by the families in the form of tisanes (teas), as they had learned to handle the various herbs and plants and understood their therapeutic value.

News that the parish priest was being transferred to Israel at the end of 1990, confirmed in May 1991, dispersed the commendable group which, with only two remaining members – Maria Muttoni and Gládis Lavarda – went back to the same places, dedicating their time to the third objective on the subject: How to cure the sick person.

This same pair of heroines also set up a fourth stage aimed at the women: culinary art, always using local produce, showing how to serve fruit and vegetables, how these can be preserved from one season to the next. This stimulated the use of sugar cane, flour milled without cylinders, beaten rice, biscuits, homemade bread and pasta, all foods no longer in use due to the more elegant-looking, refined factory-made products, often stocked on shelves in nice packaging, past their sell-by date, damaging for health, considered to be carcinogenic. In a word, their interest was to sustain the importance of homemade food, healthier and less expensive, which also helped the family finances.

Unfortunately, the situation in the parish and town hall has changed considerably. These uncertain circumstances have prevented the work from being carried out normally.

This involvement of the parish, where the parish priest is not merely a doctor of the soul, but must also treat the body, was propitious, allowing me to extend my experience with Aloe and other herbs and plants, substances that brought relief to needy people.

Q.   Are there any other remarks on Aloe, any other advice that it is worthwhile stressing before finishing the questions?

A.   Naturally, it is impossible to treat the subject of Aloe exhaustively in a few pages, but I can mention a few more facts which, in my opinion are important, without becoming too drawn-out.

1.   Aloe always and only helps the needy body; it never attacks it, it never assaults it, it never wounds it as is the case, for example, with chemotherapy. Aloe is a friend and companion. Moreover, it is your ally in the battle against disease. If at times there are effects that seem to contradict

this, you can be sure that if you continue the treatment, you will soon see that it has acted firmly, just as a doctor acts for the good of the patient or the father who punishes the child for his future good. Aloe heals the sick body instead of destroying it. After the toxic elements have been eliminated, it reintegrates the elements required to keep the body healthy. An example is the woman who had chronic intestinal problems, evidently caused by malfunctioning tissue, which doctors had been unable to cure. As I knew that Aloe cured diarrhea (Good! We are on the road to recovery!), I spoke to her about this treatment, assuring her that the unpleasant reaction (at first sight) would only last two or three days. This turned out to be the case, and the woman's problem was solved once and for all. The same thing happened to a woman with an irregular menstrual cycle. This is always the case with Aloe: it regulates blood pressure, eliminates foreign substances from the body, and normalizes cholesterol and other dysfunctions.

2. If Aloe leaves are macerated, subjected to high or low temperatures or pulverized, the curative properties of the plant are reduced. Only pick the leaves when they are required; do not keep them for long in the fridge or in any other way. Only make use of nature when in need, and it will respond according to your requirements. Prepare the blend at home; only use commercial products when you are absolutely sure they are reliable. Do not forget the

economic factor: by preparing it at home, you are helping the household finances.

3. Don't send the leaves to other regions or continents. God distributed medicinal properties in relation to the particular needs of the place, the people and the animals that make use of these plants and herbs for personalized treatment. In this way, I believe the same type of Aloe that has evolved in Palestine, Israel, the northeast of Brazil, the south of Brazil, along the Mediterranean, in Argentina, Mexico, and in the heart of Africa will undoubtedly have small but significant differences, typical of the region, without any change in its essence. Just as a cow of the same breed raised in the pampas, in Holland or in Australia will always produce milk, when this product is analyzed, there will be small differences caused by the fodder, climate, water and other factors, although it will always be milk. It is evident that the climate, the quality of the soil and atmospheric changes in the region all contribute to providing the plant with particular specifications without damaging its essence.

4. Those suffering from cancer should avoid eating meat of any type and other animal products while taking the Aloe treatment. The reason for this is simple. Cancer lives like a parasite in beings made of meat. Let's imagine that the preparation causes effects similar to those caused by food that is rotten or past its best in the stomach. By eating meat, the person with cancer "does it the favor" of helping

the ailment or disorder by bringing it a lenitive! Had you not decided to get rid of this dreadful parasite? The sick person immediately asks: "What should I eat? Just when I'm feeling so weak, I must do without meat, the most important food. Should I go hungry?"

Of course not. Meat is not essential to the human being, even those with anemia. Observation of our teeth shows that man only has two canines in each jaw (with which meat is torn) which separate four incisors (for cutting leaves and fruit), four premolars and six molars (for grinding or shredding cereals, roots, etc.). If man needed meat so badly, God would surely have given him more canines to tear the meat fibers. Cereals, fruit, vegetables and grains replace meat with advantages for the health of human beings. In addition to being easier to digest, they are also easier on the pocket!

5. Perhaps this has already been mentioned but, for clarity's sake, I think it is better to go over it once more, to explain the subject better. Our health will benefit if we do not smoke, drink or take drugs. It is said that cigarettes and alcohol provide the tax department with an income through the taxes applied. Let us imagine that the federal government collects about four billion reais (Brazilian currency) from taxes on cigarettes and alcohol. It is a fact, set down in black and white, that the government spends double this amount for diseases caused by smoking and alcohol. This system does not heal the damage caused by

smoking and alcohol, but merely treats it. Just imagine if drugs also become legalized! And that's not all. Smoking, drinking and taking drugs causes permanent damage of various kinds, lesions that not even God can heal.

Make sure that foods, especially grains, fruit and vegetables, are grown without pesticides and chemical fertilizers, even if they do not have a nice appearance. Avoid drinks with preservatives considered carcinogenic (why not prepare a freshly squeezed lemon juice, blend fruit or grains in place of traditional soft drinks?). Support and promote campaigns that seek to improve the quality of the air. Keep on demanding that industries that pollute the air use filters. Keep on demanding that industries manufacture machines or other consumer goods without polluting (technology is capable of producing motor vehicles, with the seven sisters' permission, that don't pollute!). Contribute toward introducing healthy eating habits, providing public opinion with explanations, using mass communication means, involving individuals, society, the government and the entire world and making them take action. We must collaborate for the health of human-kind. In other words "Prevention is better than the cure." It is useless to totally cleanse the body just to intoxicate it again tomorrow or the next day. It would be like cleaning out the pigsty.

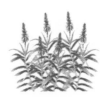

Q.　**Why are you obsessed with the idea of revealing this recipe?**

A.　Above all is the human aspect. I was with my father during the last days of his life. He had lung cancer (a smoker from the age of 14) and screamed with pain like a wounded animal, without the possibility of receiving any relief for his pain. Powerless in the face of this anguish, I asked myself a question: With all the progress modern science has made, why has it not been able to discover a remedy for this dreadful disease that inevitably leads to death? Although my father was only 63, the disease in his lungs predicted his death. He was a strong man who until then had always been fine and healthy who, nonetheless, just as all those with this disease, died unavoidably just eight months after the tumor was diagnosed.

My soul searched for the answer to the secret of this unsolvable mystery: there must be an animal, plant, mineral or something else that can solve this problem. Thankfully, about ten years later, I found the answer to my dilemma, which has become the topic of this book.

1. Because, owing to the lack of Social Security, the Brazilian health service has broken down.

2. Because official medicine has become inaccessible to over 70% of the population, which lives with extremely low incomes, a global disgrace. There is no way for looking after health, as incomes do not even cover food require-

ments. Taking care of one's health has become a luxury; the subject of health has been deleted from the list of primary needs.

3. Human life has no price, whoever and wherever the person. To save or extend a life, improving conditions is enthralling; it feels almost blissful. That is the way I felt one Sunday afternoon when I received a phone call from Cruz Alta-RS, from the mother of a girl suffering from lupus who, after just three weeks of treatment, was freed of the disease. According to her dermatologist from Ijui, the disease was incurable and the young girl would have to learn to live with it for the rest of her life. Just imagine the joyful atmosphere in the family! I am sure thousands of families have felt this same joy thanks to this simple, cheap and, in many cases, efficacious recipe.

4. The sick person I saved inexplicably becomes the child I never had, the child I relinquished in full possession of my faculties in order to dedicate all my time and energy to serving the Kingdom of God and the Brothers, whether they are Christians, Muslims, Jews, Buddhists, men or women, old or young, white or colored, rich or poor.

Beyond appearance, what is important is that they are human beings, all created in the image of God, with the right to live a WORTHY and healthy life. They are creatures to whom God reveals all his love. Many times, the majority of humans cannot even have the minimum they require to live. This is not God's fault because He did not divide things equally. It is the fault of the greed and selfishness of the strongest and most cunning, who arrogantly exploit the weak and defenseless. Good grief! We run the risk of taking the Lord's name in vain: why does God, who can do everything, not put an end to this wicked race?

In fact, by proving the marvelous effects of the recipe with various sick people who had followed their doctor's orders to the letter without obtaining any relief and who were destined to die, I started to believe in the recipe. From this point, it took just one step to reach the launching platform. I was determined to reveal the recipe, almost obstinately, especially in view of its effectiveness in solving problems considered by orthodox medicine to be incurable. The outcome of this course of action is this modest book, which I hope will help someone in difficulty or who has given up all hope.

I have had the joy of seeing tangible results with my own eyes, confirmed by the patients' families and, above all, by medical tests – definite solutions to the problem – considered a lost cause if ordinary procedures had been followed.

Is it now clear why I travel from town to town, talking to people, reaching out to them over the radio and television, without obtaining anything in return? There is no mystery! It is all very simple, just as water runs down-hill: all this can save lives.

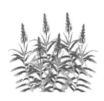

Father Romano Zago, OFM

Q. **Which countries have studied Aloe vera bardadensis the most as a medicinal plant?**

A. I believe the United States and also Russia are far ahead in this race, followed by the Japanese. On the other hand, after the atomic bombs of 50 years ago, the Japanese used Aloe widely to help people affected by the radiation produced by these diabolic weapons. Aloe reacted extremely well, so much so that some people who visited this country told me that they saw Aloe plants in many houses and flats, as it is considered the plant that heals all. Germany, Switzerland, Italy and other countries use homeopathy, which comprises Aloe. Constant work is carried out in laboratories, where the plant is dried and where new aspects are continually being discovered. These are a surprise for everyone, as its abundance cannot be measured.

Q. **As Aloe does not always have a 100% success rate in the battle against cancer, do you know of any alternatives to combat the disease, excluding orthodox medicine?**

A. Aloe does not always cure cancer, and in my travels I have come across other forms of treatment of the disease. Some of these are:

  1. **Avelco (Aveloz).** A plant from the euphorbiaceous families (scientific name: Euphorbia tirucallis), origin-

nating in Africa and mainly grown in the northeast of Brazil (see **Aurelio Dictionary**, 1ˢᵗ ed.). The promulgator of the plant, who was healed of a pleural fistula, Father Raymundo C. Welzenmann, S.J., is considered an authority in the application of the medication. For further information, contact the Padre Reus bookshop, Duque de Caxias, 805 – Porto Alegre – RS.

2. **Apple.** In Tel Aviv, Israel, there is a rabbi who treats those suffering from cancer by advising them to eat only apples. I once read in an old medical encyclopedia that eating an indefinite number of apples for a certain period of time would result in complete renewal of the blood. Could these two things be related?

3. **Honey.** Use in abundance, especially on an empty stomach, as it has strong powers of cicatrisation (healing) and preservation of the body.

4. **Water.** Dr. Aldo Alessiani of Rome applies a preparation based on water. He prefers to treat cases of cancer in the terminal phase. I personally believe that, with the advance of homeopathy, even the most serious diseases will soon be able to be cured using mere water as raw material. We shall see.

5. **Marcherium.** Extracted from our angico, and Aspidos, extracted from the pauperieira, these two Brazilian trees are considered to have anti-cancer properties. Paupereira is blind like the chemotherapy used in

traditional medicine as a therapy against cancer: Aspidos eliminates dead and diseased cells, subsequently attacking the healthy ones, with the same effect as chemotherapy. This is where Marcherium comes into play; it attempts to neutralize and rebuild the ecological disaster produced by its colleague Aspidos. Credit for this treatment goes to Silvio Rossi of Turin.

6.   **Urine.** The raw material is one's own urine. The promoters of urine therapy guarantee that this method cures cancer in three weeks. It is said it also cures AIDS.

7.   **Rattlesnake meat.** This method was learned from the Indios. They provoked the snake until it was ready to strike, the moment in which the poison is distributed evenly throughout the body. At this point, the animal is killed, the head and tail cut off, and the meat cooked over a low flame. It is then chopped finely and put into capsules, like those used for antibiotics. The patient takes a capsule before the three main meals. In Mexico it is possible to purchase capsules with rattlesnake meat in the health food shops. There is no shortage of snakes in that part of the world.

8.   **Oleander.** I received this recipe from a Palestinian lady who lives in West Bank. Using a little English, French and Arab, I managed to get the recipe from her mouth: boil four leaves from the plant in one liter

of water for 15 minutes. Take two tablespoonfuls before meals.

9. **Ipe Viola.** This tree has appeared in the last few years. In actual fact, the active ingredient against cancer is found in its bark and only in fully grown trees of about 50 years old.

10. **Mud uncontaminated by pesticides.** Applied to the affected part, it draws out many diseases, including cancer, from the body.

11. **Mucurum.** This is a blood red ornamental plant. A tisane made from its leaves in a cup of water is drunk. If the cancer is external, the boiled leaf is applied to the wound.

12. **Vitamin C.** Paul Heber of Paranapanema, Saó Paulo, Brazil, developed a product sold in capsules, based on vitamin C, which has cured cases of cancer.

I wish to stress that none of the above methods has been tested by me. My experience is based on Aloe, as it is an element that nourishes the body.

Disease is a sure sign the body is not in optimum condition. You can treat it with allopathy, homeopathy, isopathy, etc. The Aloe treatment comes under phyto-therapathy, a method known of for thousands of years throughout the world. In nature, there is indubitably the right cure for any type of disease. All we have to do is find it.

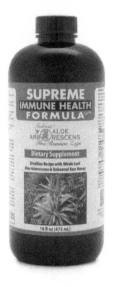

Commercial production of the Aloe Arborescens Brazilian formula for Supreme Immune Health is manufactured in North America and in Europe as a dietary supplement and distributed by health care professionals and health care product distributors.

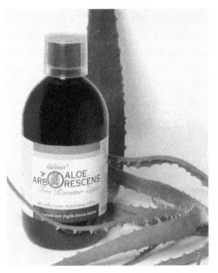

For more information on the Brazilian Supreme Immune Health Formula and the scientific papers and medical research abstracts on the properties of this aloe species, go to aloearborescens.org

Internationalization of the Recipe

In Brazil, there have been few opportunities to distribute the recipe learned in Rio Grande. Naturally, I disclosed it each time I was able to do so, by word of mouth or by letter, in the attempt to reach as many people as possible. Only once was I able to take part in Heron de Oliviera's live program on Lajeado Independent Radio. This modest diffusion has had consequences in the region of Rio Grande do Sul, Santa Catarina, in Parana, in Sao Paulo and in Minas Gerais, although to no great extent. It has perhaps reached one person in a million.

The Brazilian recipe of the Aloe, honey and distillate preparation has become universal, starting out in Israel, where I went to live in May 1991.

True progress towards internationalization of the recipe took place almost three years after I arrived in this country, after a series of healings that occurred there. However, in this phase, the recipe was still distributed through interpersonal relations.

At the international level, diffusion of the recipe commenced in November-December 1993 through an article in the magazine **The Holy Land** by Vittorio Bosello, OFM, published in Italian, Spanish (with supplement in Portuguese), French, English and Arab, later summarized by Father Dario Pili, OFM, who also benefited from the recipe and who had surgery in the Policlinico Gemelli hospital in Rome (where Pope John Paul II had also

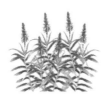

been treated on various occasions), for cancer of the throat and, according to medical tests, is totally cured.

As he attributes his cure to the benefits of this preparation, Father D. Pili wrote an extremely pleasing introduction. This introduction was used for the sister magazines.

The recipe spread throughout the five continents rapidly. Due to its importance, the news was reported by other newspapers and magazines, inasmuch as it was shouted from the rooftops that the simple preparation could cure tumors and other diseases – all proven by facts.

The stories of some healings are set out below.

- The period of four years I served at the Custody of the Holy Land in Israel started on May 7, 1991. The Jewish island between Arabs and Muslims still smelled of the dust raised by the war against Saddam Hussein's claims on Kuwait, written down in history as the Gulf War.

  After I had a month of settling in, my superiors decided to appoint me to the Holy Sepulchre, considered to be the most important Christian sanctuary in the world, as it was here that the historical event of Jesus Christ's resurrection took place. Due to the Gulf War, there were very few pilgrimages. However, in times of peace, it is filled with tourists, pilgrims and priests from the Christian West who dream of celebrating Mass in this sanctuary at least once in their lives.

- The Sacristian Brothers are always in difficulty when the usual number of pilgrims is present. They are helped by a young Arab called Issa. Immediately after the pilgrims had left, I saw the youth leaving the sacristy and going to the Arab Hospital in Jerusalem, where he was treated with some method or other. The brothers told me the boy was dying; he had a ganglion lymphoma. Having had several successes with Aloe, I offered to save the young Arab, who is still alive today. The doctors could not understand it. Who can understand? But the fact is that the boy is now 25 and continues to do his job, happily serving the pilgrims who come to visit the Holy Sepulchre to ask for the privilege to celebrate or participate in a Mass.

- The second case in which I took action, in chronological order, was the secretary of the Holy Land school in Bethlehem, Israel. On August 31, 1991, my superiors decided to transfer me from the Holy Sepulchre in Jerusalem to the birthplace of Jesus – Bethlehem – so I could teach Latin and serve as a tutor for students studying philosophy. It was in this community that the headmaster of the school was having problems with his secretary, who was extremely ill. I naturally offered my help and the secretary was totally cured and is still alive today.

- On December 12, I received a letter from Father Alviero Niccaci, OFM, the head of the Pontificale Athenaeum Antonianum in Rome, from his branch Studium Biblicum Franciscanum in Jerusalem, informing me that his Indian pupil, Father Thomas, had had surgery for brain cancer in Hadassa Hospital in Jerusalem. After the operation, he had had strange infections with enormous tumors on the head and neck, malodorous and oozing, so much so that the man had to take his meals alone. I prepared the recipe according to the formula. In a nutshell, the bronze-colored Indian was able to take his exams for the school year and return to his own country in perfect health.

I would love to report the entire content of Father Niccaci's letter. In his desperate appeal, he said, "Please help us." You can sense all the concern and anxiety of the headmaster for his disciples.

- The Lebanese Sister Muna, a sister of Saint Joseph, was headmistress of a girls' school in the Holy Land. She had urgent surgery to remove an ovary. Just two months later, the other ovary was removed. After less than two months, the doctors at Hadassa Hospital, one of the best equipped in Israel, found an enormous tumor in the womb. According to her relatives, she only had 15 days to live. I was asked to help her with Aloe. This was in 1992 and, whether you believe it or not, the sister is still alive today. She has routine tests at the hospital, which show that she has been cured, although the doctors are unable to explain how this woman is still alive and was able to return to her job as headmistress of the school.

- Sister Miriam of Bethlehem in Palestine, a Franciscan Missionary of Mary, took me aside to tell me she was worried about her nephew, a man of about 50, who along with three other Palestinian friends, had had surgery (which lasted about 12 hours) for cancer of the throat at Hadassa Hospital. She insisted that I save him, as he still had small children to look after. The worst thing was that he was unable to swallow. I devised a plan to allow him to take the preparation, the only way of saving his life. After blending it, I filtered the blend so the pulverized leaves would not clog the cannula used to feed him. In this way, he took several jars. The happy ending is that the nun's nephew moved to Jordan, where he manages properties and leads a normal life.

His three friends, who had throat surgery in the Jewish hospital without using Aloe, all died, one after another. Sister Miriam lives in St. Joseph's house, a sanctuary at the Milk Grotto.

- Sister Margherita, an Italian Franciscan Sister of the Immaculate Heart of Mary, was diagnosed with breast cancer. She had treatment in the Italian Hospital in Haifa, Israel. When I heard of her problem, I offered to prepare the compound for her. She took it and felt so good that she immediately went back to work without taking any tests. She allowed herself to be guided by her well-being, going back to her work as usual. However, inside her body the disease was still at work. One day it reared its head again. Less than a year later, the nun's soul went to God. The support of medical tests, together with the preparation, was missing. Not kept under control, the cancer came back with violence and took another of its countless victims. Sister Margherita is the most convincing example of how someone suffering from cancer must have tests and treatment, otherwise...

- In the shadow of the Nativity Church in Bethlehem, Israel, a woman of about 40 of Orthodox religion, with a family, was lying bedridden with cancer of the spinal column. I was asked to help. The lady took Aloe for one week. She got out of bed and went back to her domestic life, refusing, for some unknown reason, to continue to take the potion. It could not have been otherwise: about four months later, she died. In this case, just as for Sister Margherita, continuity and perseverance were missing.

However, there are people who wish to die. In this case, there is no medicine that can help. In these situations, psychological support is required to try to reverse the trend, to give the person new reason to live, so that healing can take place.

- A youngish woman had surgery at the Hadassa Hospital in Bethlehem, Israel, located in the shadow of the Sacred Heart Church run by the commendable Salesian Fathers. Various complications made her turn to my preparation. After four days of treatment, she was finally able to empty her bowels. Aloe is a strong laxative that regulates the bowels.

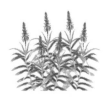

- The cousin of one of my clerics from the Lebanon, Friar Toufic, a twenty-year-old philosophy student in Bethlehem, was bedridden in his parents' home with cancer of the spinal column. He could sit up in bed with someone's help, managing to stay in this position for five minutes at the most. Fra Toufic went home on holiday at the end of the school year with a jar of Aloe in his suitcase, ready to be taken, certain that it would help his dear cousin. After finishing the jarful, the boy got up and went to visit friends and relatives, once again able to go about his business.

- In Jordan, a boy with cancer of the face, deformed through the treatment which he went regularly to the United States for, took three doses of the preparation. According to the Sisters of St. Dorothy from the Latin Patriarchate Seminary in Beit Jala, Bethlehem, the boy was cured and stopped making those expensive journeys abroad.

- A man named Andrea worked as an electrician in the enormous St. Saviour Friary, seat of the Custody of the Holy Land. He was originally from the former Yugoslavia, was extremely good at his job and was married to an Arab woman. After having worked in the monastery for many years, he was asked by the friars, against their will, to leave as he had been diagnosed with prostate cancer, which devastated him. The doctors operated on him several times, the last time removing his testicles ("to the great joy of some cats," Andrea jokes), to prevent the disease from reaching the lymphatic system of the body, which would have meant death. Andrea lived in a wheelchair, depending on his wife and friends for everything for six months. Brother Luis Garcia, who managed the monastery and with whom Andrea had had most contact due to the similarities in their jobs, having witnessed the cure of another Spanish brother, Father Carlos, who had a tumor in his head, asked me for a jar of the miraculous preparation. It provided the best result possible: Andrea was completely cured. As the brothers had already employed another electrician, thinking Andrea would never get better, they lost him to the Sisters of St. Vincent, who knew how well he worked and his easygoing nature, and didn't think twice about employing him. Andrea works in the sisters' community beside Jaffa Street in Jerusalem and no one can compete with him.

- One of the most well-known cases, so much so it can be said it influenced the world, among those narrated in the magazine **The Holy Land**, is the story of Geraldito, the Argentinian child who has returned to his country and now lives a normal life like all other children of his age.

- A case similar to Geraldito's comes to mind, this time in Nazareth, Israel. Seliman (Solomon) also had leukemia. According to the doctors, Seliman required a bone marrow transplant, which was impossible as no donors had been found. Although the boy had two brothers, neither of them was compatible. His father was a doctor and, taking advantage of his connections with the medical category, he advertised for donors in publications, even in the United States. When I heard of Geraldito, I told Seliman's mother, Maria, that I hoped no donor would be found, because if he were to take the Aloe, honey and distillate preparation, he would not need one. The child started taking the preparation three years ago and has always managed to get through the school year. At the end of another school year, before Seliman's family left to spend their summer holidays in Italy, Maria phoned me to tell me happily that her son had been first in his class that year. I wished her happy holidays and a safe journey home and continued to hope that no donor would be found. If taken regularly now and again, the Aloe would keep the child healthy.

We now leave Israel and the surrounding area to look at other cases of people who have been cured.

- A phone call from Bangkok in Thailand informed me that the Salesian priest Don Personini of Bergamo, Italy, a missionary in this Asian country, had ordered Aloe for his mother after reading the magazine **The Holy Land**, last edition of 1993, November-December. As a result, his mother was cured. He was so enthusiastic over the Aloe that he sent a person of his trust to Bethlehem in Israel to identify the plant and take the preparation ready for use to a boy suffering from leukemia. Father Personini sent the recipe from the magazine to his sister in Bergamo, who was looking after their sick mother. I was informed of the final result in a letter sent to me in Bethlehem.

- A few weeks later I had a visit from another Salesian brother who had studied in Bethlehem at the International Institute of Theology in Cremisan. The family involved in this problem had financed his journey, and he had covered a distance of 15,000 kilometers (9,300 miles) to learn the secret of the potion and take several doses ready for use away in his suitcase. The priest, who also performed apostolic work in Korea, assured me he would take the secret there, too. While passing through Europe on his way back, he visited the home of his fellow brother's mother, now totally cured, in Bergamo.

- Through the editorial office of **The Holy Land**, I received a letter in French, informing me that Alla, a 12-year-old girl, had been affected by radiation following the Chernobyl nuclear disaster. After just one month of treatment with the preparation, the girl returned to Kiev in the Ukraine, totally cured. The way in which Alla was cured is remarkable: an oncologist from Moscow in Russia sent a letter to France, where Alla was on holiday, asking that the girl be treated with Father Romano Zago's recipe. How did the oncologist hear of the recipe? Had he used the recipe on others affected by radioactivity? Why not use it on all Chernobyl victims?

- Rosita G. from Ticino in Switzerland who, according to the doctors, only had three months to live, had cancer of the liver, pancreas and spleen. They forecast that in the last stage of the disease, her pain would be so great that her screams would send everyone running. She took various jars of the preparation. She needed no painkillers. She took no type of chemical medicines. She died at eighty, without any pain, conscious and lucid, like a candle burning out.

- The archbishop of Belgrade wrote to Josephine in Switzerland. Because he had brain cancer, he was unable even to sign cards at Christmas. Now, after taking the Aloe treatment, he has left the hospital and gone to live in the home for retired priests. He is no longer blind and he can read the paper. The letters Josephine receives are written directly by him.

- According to Soeur Isabelle, the contemplative sisters of the Notre-Dame de l'Assomption Convent in Beth Gemal, Betshemesh in Israel have always had success with the jars of preparation sent to France and Belgium, from where most of them come. All the doses have had 100% success rates, with no exceptions.

- Sister Lisette, from the Santana Church in Jerusalem, came to visit me to thank me for the healing of the Dutch missionary, Van Ass, of the White Priests, who was suffering from cancer of the liver. The doctors had given him only three months to live and the missionary had consequently left his work in Africa to die in his own country of Holland so he could make use of the resources a developed country can offer its citizens. Sister Lisette was unable to tell me how many doses of Aloe Van Ass had taken, but she assured me that the missionary had gone back happily to the Black Continent, where he has been in perfect health for over a year.

- Ida called me from the Venice Lido in Italy. She told me that her sister Silvana's husband, Giampaolo B., had had surgery for a tumor of the cerebellum. During a checkup by the doctor who had performed the surgery, she had witnessed the great surprise of the surgeon, who was incredulous over the success of such a delicate operation. The doctor was so pleased over the man's condition that he made the next appointment for a next check-up seven months later. The patient, who had been unable to do anything for himself, has now returned to work, drives the car, eats and sleeps; in other words, he leads a normal life. Imagine my surprise when I received a phone call telling me that all three would be disembarking from a ship in the port of Haifa in Israel, with their own car driven by Giampaolo himself, to express their thanks in person at the Nativity Monastery where I was then staying!

- Mrs. Evelina B., from Florence, Italy, told me that her sister Teresa, suffering from bone cancer and confined to a wheelchair, had recently felt that her strength was returning. Subsequently, when I went to visit her in 1995, I found Teresa an active housewife moving freely around the house without requiring a cane, going about her work with good color and a happy smile. As gratitude for the healing that occurred, the family asked me to send the measurements of the crib of the manger in Bethlehem, as they wish to make a cradle in worked gold for the Baby Jesus of the Grotto.

- Father Vincente Ianello, OFM, who is the keeper of the Convent of the Flagellation in Jerusalem, Israel, is overjoyed. His sister from the Naples area works miracles using Father Romano Zago's recipe. It has healed a lady with brain cancer, another with cancer of the throat, and a man with bone cancer. She is currently treating a child with brain cancer.

- Received a telephone call from the father of Luciano M., a 15-month-old child. The doctors said they had only seen one other case like his before, which in any case was incurable. After the treatment, Luciano was examined. According to the doctors, the child no longer had any traces of cancerous cells! When they went to the child's room to tell his mother, she couldn't hold back the tears of joy – he had been born again! His father, radiant, told me he had carefully kept all the papers and they were at my disposal. He also said he didn't know whether to believe it, as it was too good to be true!

- Sister Carla, General Mother of the Sisters of the Heart of Jesus, visited me in Bethlehem, together with her secretary, to thank me for having been healed of breast cancer. She had asked for and received a jar of the preparation.

- Micol, a 13-year-old who lives near Ancona in Italy, had had brain cancer since she was five. She has had three surgeries at the Oncological Centre in Paris, perhaps the most famous in the world. However, the Beast came back with double the strength. No cortisone or morphine could calm the pain. A fourth operation was not possible. After taking a jar of the Aloe treatment, the child was no longer in pain. She could ride her bike, play and talk. However, tests showed that the disease was still spreading through her body. After taking a second dose, the results of another cycle of tests were completely different. There was no longer any trace of the disease – how marvelous!

- Rita and Paolo's three-year-old daughter, Carolina, from Florence in Italy, has leukemia. Although in the hospital to have chemotherapy, she took a jar of the preparation. Her test values decreased from 70% to 30%. The doctors explained these results to her parents in the following way: Before the treatment there was a kind of desert in Carolina's body. Now her body is filled with flora, scattered here and there, and the symptoms of the disease seem to have decreased. The latest news is that Carolina is well. In gratitude for her healing, Paolo and Rita have decided to adopt another child.

- Father Lorenzo, Conventual OFM from Parma, had cancer of the colon. The doctors opened his lower stomach but could do nothing. Before closing him up, they decided by mutual consent to perform a colostomy, to give him the chance, depending on how well he recovered, to have some radiotherapy and chemotherapy in an attempt to prolong his life. However, Father Lorenzo has a guardian angel who immediately started to prepare the Aloe blend for him. To sum up, just three months after the operation, Father Lorenzo's health was so good that the doctors who operated the first time removed the sack they had applied. So Father Lorenzo is once again as God created him. The priest currently lives his 70 years of age smiling and happy, sought after throughout the world as a charismatic confessor, much loved in his country. His is another case among many who, after having had a colostomy, returned to their former condition.

- Gregorio from Milan in Italy had a tumor of 9 cm in the bladder. The doctors in Como were preparing to operate. They couldn't decide whether to remove the bladder and replace it with a plastic one or leave him without a bladder. Gregorio was afraid and phoned me to ask for help. After one jar of Aloe, the tumor had decreased from 9 to 2 cm. After a second jar, Gregorio's tumor disappeared. The doctors from Como were astounded! Gregorio lives his life with the bladder God gave him. He came to the conference I held in Milan one Sunday afternoon, happy to be alive, to tell everyone about his experience.

- Six-year-old Christopher suffered from leukemia and went to Bethlehem with his parents Joaquim Eugenio and Fatima to see the doctors, who gave him just two months to live. But that was before he took Aloe. From being confined to a wheelchair, he became as free as a bird without having to depend on anyone, although he dragged his right leg slightly. Two weeks after a second dose taken in Bethlehem, his father telephoned me to inform me that the two-month period had passed. Also, the child no longer dragged his leg and was no longer anemic. The couple tried to convince me to go to Mozambique and South Africa to publicize the recipe and help people there. Joaquim Eugenio Ferraz and his family live in Pretoria. Before returning home, Christopher gave me a Seiko watch to remember him by as, in his opinion, I am responsible for his healing. In truth, he was cured thanks to Aloe and its preparation.

- Miriam, a Jewish woman who lives in Jerusalem, heard of the effects of Aloe. She invited me to her home for me to teach her the secret. She lent me her apron so that I would not soil my Franciscan frock. Before her eyes I prepared two doses, one for her and one for her husband. She wanted to try it out on herself. After the first jar, Miriam became a promoter of the Aloe preparation among friends and acquaintances, both in Israel and Italy. She has experienced the joy of curing many brothers. Miriam has a true veneration for Franciscans, as during the Second World War and the persecution of the Jews, Father Riccardo Niccaci in Assisi saved her family by hiding them in the attic of the convent, away from the anti-Semitic attacks. One thing is sure: the Aloe, honey and distillate preparation is in use among the Jews.

- In the Biology Department of Hadassa Hospital in Jerusalem, it is possible to receive treatment with the potion. It was there that Sister Muna, a patient in the hospital, heard the doctors treating her say, "How marvelous Father Romano's cure is!" This preparation, associated with therapeutic mud from the Dead Sea (Sodom and Gomorrah) is also available in hotels that receive guests affected by skin diseases (lupus, psoriasis, etc.) considered incurable by traditional medicine.

- At Santo Antonio Hospital in Porto, Portugal, everyone suffering from cancer can have the Aloe, honey and distillate preparation if they wish.

- Before any other therapy, Dr. Enza Capaci from Palermo in Sicily, Italy, advises any patients suffering from cancer to take one or two doses of the Aloe, honey and distillate potion. She says that, to date, the Aloe has always had a beneficial effect, even if modest, such as alleviating pain.

- Ruggero telephoned me from Ravenna in Italy on February 24, 1994 to tell me he had cancer of the vocal chords. He asked me to send him a jar of honey ready for use. The jar was sent urgently, as he was rapidly losing his voice. On May 20, 1994, I was happy to receive another call from Ruggero informing me that his voice was back to normal (in fact, everything was back to normal). Tests showed that the cancer had disappeared!

- Sister Emilia Birck, F.D.C., from Rio Grande do Sul, who was working in England, wrote to tell me that the young P.E. teacher in her school had had to resign as she was suffering from cancer. I wrote back immediately, telling her to use the preparation without delay. It could have been no different: the young teacher is already back at work.

- In July 1995, Brother Bernardo Kleinert, OFM, had an operation that removed the phalanx of the second toe of his left foot. In November of the same year, he lost the big toe of the same foot. An X-ray showed that he had acute osteomyelitis, made worse by his diabetes.

On January 4, 1996, the Father Superior of the Province, Father Nestor Inacio Schwerz, was asked to write a document on behalf of the Order and Brother Bernardo's family, authorizing the doctors to amputate the brother's leg from the knee down to prevent gangrene from spreading. The area that had been operated on previously had extensive necrosis, with poor circulation and total lack of sensitivity. Brother Bernardo was 1.93 m (6'3") tall and weighed 77 kg (170 lbs.).

Still in the first week of January, 1996, the doctors were asked to wait before amputating. He then started to take the Aloe cure. He took it both orally and it was applied to the skin, alternated with canary grass tisanes, doses of mallow, walnut, artichoke and, after meals, magnesium chloride.

After taking the content of the first bottle for fifteen days, the wound had decreased by 50%. Blood was once again reaching the area of the first operation, which was thus oxygenated. Circulation and sensitivity returned, all without the aid of any chemical drugs. On March 22, 1996, another X-ray was taken at the Divina Providencia Hospital in Porto Alegre. Dr. Mauro T. Master interpreted the exam by comparing it to the previous X-rays. His verdict was "almost certain total regression of the signs of osteomyelitis in the first metatarsus. No other changes." The results of the last X-ray on September 25, 1996, taken in the same hospital and interpreted by the same doctor were "there has been resection of the distal segment of the 1st metatarsus. The edema of the soft parts of the foot has regressed. No other changes."

Today the wound is nothing but a scar. At the beginning of October, 1996, Brother Bernardo returned to the Sao Boraventura Convent in Daltro Filho, Imigrante, to resume his normal everyday activities after eight months of treatment with Aloe, having regained his normal weight and with diabetic values of 85-95, against a maximum tolerable value of 110.

- The youngest son of Antonia V. F. from Grancona Vicenza in Italy had sudden attacks of vomiting and unconsciousness, possibly the sign of some inner instability. Matteo had always been a normal child. After several tests in Verona, the doctors found two foci in the brain and a cyst. You can imagine how worried Antonia was! On her own initiative, she gave the preparation to the child without following the indications too strictly, as he was at nursery school and couldn't take the lunchtime dose, there being no one in the school who could give it to him. After a few months of treatment, Antonia went back to Verona for more tests and a medical examination. The doctors were amazed when they found the two foci and the cyst had disappeared. This diagnosis was confirmed by an encephalogram and CAT scan.

I could go on and on for many more pages, case after case. If readers wish to know more, they can refer to the notes I took during four years of work in Israel. Almost every day I recorded some new fact, many times also noting down the name, address and telephone number of the person who had been cured.

Plant an Aloe arborescens shoot; this will give you a complete pharmacy, which God places at your disposal.

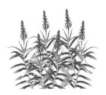

The Composition of Aloe Vera or Barbadensis

The world has known about Aloe for thousands of years, and it has gone down in the history of a wide variety of cultures and civilizations as the plant of myth and magic, used also as a medicinal plant, but without scientific backing. The use of Aloe for therapeutic purposes is described in various medical journals from the 2nd Century A.D. to the 17th Century, although chemical analyses on organic material were virtually unknown until the 19th Century. Only in 1851 was the bitter, dark viscous substance extracted from Aloe crystallized and identified as Aloin (see **Silent Healer**, p. 65). It was classified as a cathartic and its pharmacological use started to take on the same importance it had already had primitively. Although its curative properties were known, the plant still had folkloristic or mystical connotations.

From 1930 on, many scholars have dedicated their studies to the plant by sectioning it and analyzing it, inside and out.

Collins and Crewe in the 1930s were the first to use the plant professionally. They successfully treated skin burns caused by radioactivity. This was to be the beginning of a long haul, with the objective of revealing the extraordinary qualities of Aloe.

In 1938, Chopia and Gosh identified the principal components of the plant: emodin, aloin, chrysophanic acid, resin, rubber, and

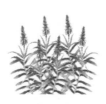

volatile and non-volatile traces of acid – an important collaboration.

However, it was only in 1941, thanks to the efforts of Prof. D. Rowe, that Aloe received its first detailed description. With tireless dedication in searching for the truth and through chemical analysis of the plant, Prof. Rowe was able to give it credibility.

Tom D. Rowe and Lloyd M. Parks performed in-depth analysis of the plant and recorded their results in the newspaper of the American Pharmaceutical Association.

Other names of great scientists could be added to the list, although we shall possibly omit some important names. Those we particularly remember are:

Gottshall, Lorenzetti, Maria Luisa D'Amico, G.A. Bravo, Icawa, Niemann, El Zawahry, Hegazy, Helal, Gumar Gjerstad, G. D. Bouchey, Ruth Sims, E. R. Zimmermann, Kenichi Imanishi, T. E. Danhof, Fujita, H. Tsuda, K. Matsumoto, M. Ito and I. Hirono, among others.

Each one made an important contribution to complete the knowledge of this wonder of nature.

Without going into the merits of the studies of each scientist, after 20 years of intense work, what have they found in Aloe that is useful for humans and animals?

1.   Lignin: a substance similar to pulp, existing in a formation with cellulose and of which the gel of the Aloe leaf is made up. It penetrates human skin extremely well. Its medicinal properties are currently unknown.

2.   Saponin: these are glycosides that do not merely have antiseptic and cleansing properties; they are also superb saponaceous agents used in cosmetics such as shampoo.

3.   Anthraquinone compound: this is a laxative agent known to be a formidable exterminator of diseases. Anthraquinone is known as a valid bactericidal agent, in line with traditional antibiotics, but with fewer toxic effects and greater anti-viral capacities.

3.1.   Aloin is a free resin, a soluble extract of Aloe. Its color varies from lemon yellow to dark yellow. It has an extremely bitter taste and turns dark upon contact with air and light. It acts as a cathartic.

3.2.   Barbaloin derives from Aloe in crystalline form. It increases the potency of the anthraquinone. It is a cathartic with spasmodic effects on the digestive tract and is considered an effective analgesic.

3.3.   Isobarbaloin: this is an isomer of barbaloin and is therefore more concentrated.

3.4.   Glycoside barbaloin: this crystalline resin is formed from Aloe. Derivatives are compound anthraquinones, anthracene and acetic acids, especially effective against pain; it has important antibiotic properties.

3.5.   Aloe-Emodin: this is a yellow crystalline form of Aloe. Its name is hydroxyl-methylanthraquinone. Known for its laxative effect, it has certain anti-infection qualities in relation to many anthraquinones. When subjected individually to tests to identify their capacities to inhibit Staphylococcus aureus, Aloe-emodin and emodin failed; when tested together with the gel of the leaf, they turned out to be bactericides against a vast range of bacteria.

3.6.   Aloetic acid: its technical reference is hydroxymethyl-anthraquinone, aloetic acid and Aloe purpura. It derives from Aloe-emodin. Its actual contributions toward healing are unknown, except those of compound anthraquinone.

3.7.   Ether oil: the liquid extract, when compared to ether oil, contains many anesthetic and analgesic properties already found in ether, apart from its specific toxicity.

3.8.   Chrysophanic acid: the methylanthraquinone derived from Aloe-emodin is known for its effective treatment of chronic skin diseases, such as psoriasis and trichophytosis.

3.9. Cinnamic acid: this is in relation to cinnamon compounds and has important carminative and digestive activity; this acid is considered useful as a germicide, fungicide, and detergent.

3.10. Ester of cinnamic acid: this is a hydrolyzing and proteolitic enzyme, produced by the action of cinnamic acid in the body. This perpetuates enzymatic decomposition of the tissue in necrosis and may act as an analgesic.

3.11. Resistannol: the alcohol derives from cinnamic acids and interacts with these. Resistannol is considered a carrier of certain bactericide capacities, although separate testing does not prove this.

4.   Inorganic components and minerals: these are classified as mineral elements of the human body. They are harmful when

too many or too few. They interact with certain vitamins, co-enzymes and proteolytic enzymes.

4.1. Calcium: Known to be an essential element for the human body. Perhaps comparable to iron, it is especially required to develop bone tissue in the young or to regenerate damaged tissue. It is in direct relation to phosphorus. Excess calcium in the body can cause bone deformities, calcified deposits and tissue hardening. The lack of calcium causes weak bone formation. Its importance in the reconstruction of tissue is immeasurable.

4.2. Sodium, potassium and chlorine: these are fundamental salts in the body and are closely linked to each other. Sodium and potassium are particularly important for the human body as they are essential for regulating metabolism. Potassium salts are essential elements to facilitate muscle extension and contraction, to retain water, and for the chemical balance of the body. Sodium is fundamental to maintain the correct degree of water; it is especially important in the regulation of adult metabolism and is also required to stabilize adrenaline hormones, such as aldosterone. Chlorine is less significant, as there is no established minimum quantity, but it is important to form sodium chloride and potassium and in other chloride combinations. The three elements are essential to regulate the flow of other elements in the chemistry of the body and facilitate the natural flow of the healing process. Lack of these minerals may cause damage to the body. Lack of potassium can cause muscular contractions (cramps), dizziness, and even temporary blindness. Lack of sodium can cause considerable energy loss, nausea, and serious metabolic problems. Too much chlorine may cause a toxic reaction and create specific infections. High blood pressure and cardiovascular problems can be caused by excess sodium in the body.

4.3. Zinc: this is perhaps the most widely used mineral. There is no minimum nutritional value established for zinc in the body, although there is an established level of importance. It is closely associated with food proteins and is prevalent in some types of natural grain and fish. Dysfunctions caused by zinc deficiency are anemia and hypo-glandular problems. Recent studies indicate that zinc is directly related to sexual potency and genital-urinary problems. In most men, prostatitis is caused by a zinc deficiency. Too much zinc inhibits the effects of other elements, especially iron.

4.4. Manganese: this is considered essential for human beings and is found in the bones, liver, pituitary, pineal and mammary glands. The lack of this element slows down growth and causes nervous disorders and infertility.

4.5. Magnesium: for its properties and chemical composition, it is in relation to manganese, although it has different functions. It is found mainly in the liver and muscular tissues. It is important for breast-feeding mothers and the development of children. Significant levels of magnesium deficiency can cause malabsorption syndrome, chronic alcoholism, excessive irritability, dilation of blood vessels and convulsions. It is directly related to calcium and potassium in regulating human metabolism.

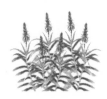

4.6. Copper. This metal element is not easily absorbed by the human body. Only 30% of copper swallowed is actually absorbed; the rest is eliminated during the evacuation process. The lack of copper in animals and humans causes problems of anemia, degeneration of the nervous system, and cardiovascular lesions.

4.7. Chromium: important for the human body, especially to activate enzymes through the synthesis of fatty acids and cholesterol. It is fixed mainly in the spleen, kidneys, testicles, heart, lungs and brain. It is found in many enzymes and RNA molecules. Without chromium, the body would be particularly susceptible to a delay in glucose tolerance and susceptible to sugar in disorders such as diabetes.

There is no evidence that Aloe contains iron or sulphuric minerals, although it contains mucopolysaccharide derivatives such as methionine, cystine, and amino acid sulphates. What is known is that there are possibly elements in the muco-polysaccharides of the gel of the leaf capable of stimulating mineral activity in the human body.

Regarding the importance of minerals as curative agents in the human body, the question is open to debate, although there is no doubt that when a body is sick or tissues are damaged, minerals are required to rebuild it. Minerals are essential in the healing process.

5. Talking about vitamins opens a debate that often becomes a subject for controversy. Each vitamin has its pros and cons. The minimum amounts have been acknowledged with a certain

degree of unanimity, although maximum levels have not yet been established. For this reason, it is believed that taking vitamins A and K in high dosages can have negative effects, such as circulation blockages and perhaps even brain damage. Vitamin B6 taken in large quantities is said to be responsible for debilitating the body. Although we now have a great deal of knowledge, we still are not sure to what extent vitamins are necessary in nourishment and what functions they have in the human body. We do not know what types of vitamins are essential for nourishment and whether they are vital for survival.

In practice, if the body becomes debilitated or gets ill, vitamins are the first elements that must be reintegrated to restore the body to health.

No one is claiming that Aloe has all the vitamins required to restore energy lost during the disease. It is claimed that certain vitamins are found in the Aloe gel. Let's have a quick look at the essential vitamins found in Aloe.

5.1. Vitamin 131: also known as thyamine or oryzamine, this works as a co-enzyme in the metabolism. It is directly linked to appetite, the growth of tissues, the digestion, nervous activities, and energy production. Its absence causes edema and neuritis.

5.2. Niacinamide (niacin): this is an enzymatic combination of nicotinic acid and tryptophanic enzymes. Its nutritional power is important, even essential, for the body, not just to compensate for a co-enzymatic agent against diseases and dermatitis, but also because, being a source of basic energy, it also compensates for the metabolic agents hydrogen and choline.

5.3. Vitamin B2: better known as riboflavin, it works as a co-enzyme in the respiratory system. It is the primary element of the condiment proteins, essential for the health and treatment of the skin, to reduce oxidation of the system and tissue of the eye. It is the principal agent to renew blood, and lack of it can cause anemia.

5.4. Vitamin B6: better known as pyridoxine, this is a co-enzyme in many phases of the metabolism of amino acids and is essential for the development of growth. It is the life-giving vitamin. Although its interactive properties in the regeneration of tissues cannot be measured, it cannot be denied that it is important for the structure of amino acids in the body.

5.5. Vitamin C (ascorbic acid): probably the best known vitamin in the world, it is part of the Aloe complex. It is known for its preventive action against disease. In high and regular doses, it has a preventive action on colds and streptococcal infections and has become the most widely used cure in the world for catarrh and influenza. Some scientists dispute these findings, as they have not been confirmed by tests. It is certain that it is a catalyst for the human body, increasing the level of tolerance to colds and flu, and also functions in the metabolism of enzymes, helping in the growth of tissues, to heal wounds, synthesize polysaccharides, and form collagen. It combats infections and is essential for the formation of bones and teeth.

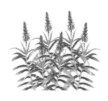

5.6. Vitamin E: in pharmacology, Vitamin E belongs to the tocopherol family, synthesized as a-tocopherol. It has been acknowledged as factor x. This vitamin is perhaps the least known aspect of Aloe. It is important to the health of skin, growth of tissues, especially those that require maximum efficiency of fatty acids, and organs such as the liver, kidneys, intestine and genitals. It promotes healthy production of bone marrow and healthy tissue. Lack of it can cause skin problems, anemia, and bone deformities. In high doses it helps eliminate infections. It is used topically and internally to treat patients with burns. There is catalogued data proving its efficacy against carcinogenic agents found in the tar of cigarettes and in toxic gases such as nitrites. For many years, it has been considered efficacious in respiratory problems, pneumonia and asthma. It protects fatty acids by absorbing them and helping them to convert rapidly into proteins so they can help combat diseases. It is found in large quantities in the gel of Aloe leaves in the form of tocopherol oxide.

5.7. Choline is still an enigma in the human body. It belongs to the group of B complex vitamins, but does not act alone. It works well with vitamin E, especially in the metabolism of fatty tissues and enzymatic activities. It prevents disorders of the liver and kidneys, as it is essential in tissue regeneration.

5.8. Folic acid is another vitamin that works better in combination with others, particularly those from group B. It is stimulated by ascorbic acid (vitamin C), which allows it to parti-cipate in enzymatic activities. Folic acid has been considered extremely useful in the structure of blood and in combating anemia.

It must be stressed that the vitamin content of Aloe, for all vitamins and minerals present, complies with the minimum doses required in daily use. Technology and medicine have the task of completing what is missing in the plant when dealing with a body with deficiencies. Even if some vitamins and mineral salts are only present in small quantities, the importance that some of these have on others and on the enzymatic activities in the body is acknowledged. According to commonly recognized scientific measurements, vitamins and mineral salts may not have a particular significance in the healing process. The majority of vitamins gave no positive results in laboratory tests performed separately. However, it is important to consider the ingredients collectively.

Therefore, is there an active ingredient that can reveal the mystery of Aloe so its reliability can be fixed objectively and its credibility as a medicinal plant is no longer disputed? The answer is that the active ingredient acts through synergism. The exact meaning of synergism is "the working together of one or more agents to produce an effect greater than the sum of their individual effects." When we understand this principle, it is obvious that many elements with considerable therapeutic potential, considered essential to the vital process in a healthy body, when taken separately are, in most cases, unsuccessful or produce doubtful results.

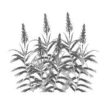

Up to this point, it seems evident that many anthraquinone compounds of minerals and vitamins, when used synergistically, have exciting effects that cannot be observed in the laboratory. This concept of synergism cannot be stressed enough in understanding the components of Aloe. It is the combination that makes the plant perfect. The problem with tests is that they don't tell the whole story, and this may not meet the expectations of the theory, leading to the conclusion that the combination is ineffective.

6.   The mucopolysaccharides identified in Aloe are cellulose-glucose, mannose, uronic acid, aldonentose and L-rhamnose.

7.   The enzymes (comprising the great proteolytic complexes) identified in the Aloe gel are oxidase, catalase, amylase, cellulase and aliinase.

8.   The amino acids identified in the Aloe gel are: lysine, threonine, valine, thionin, leucine, isoleucine, phenyalanine, histidine, arginine, hydroxyproline, cuparatic acid, serine, glutammic acid, proline, glycerine, alanine, cystine and tyrosine.

This list may seem excessively long, although in truth it should be much longer, as there are only five enzymes in it.

By observing the result of reducing sugars and amino acids, we can presume that there are at least another twenty or thirty enzymes. According to the latest estimates, about 900 enzymes have been identified in the human body, although there are many more.

In the case of amino acids, the situation is more complicated. There are 22 amino acids in the healthy body. Eight of these are considered essential, as they are made by the body starting from eight essential amino acids. In Aloe, we find 20 of the 22 amino acids and also seven of the eight considered essential. The eighth, tryptophan, which it seems has never been identified, is known to be a component of the niacinamide complex; it is highly likely that this is found in Aloe. The probability of its existence is so likely that the presence of the amino acid complex in Aloe appears to be complete. Moreover, these amino acids can make an enormous number of combinations. I have attempted to give an example of the great healing potential found in Aloe.

The part these elements play in healing body diseases can be appreciated only after we have understood the body's basic needs. First, the body is composed of a great number of chemical products, the most important of which, for life and health, are proteins. The protein molecule is formed of 20 different compounds called amino acids, used to provide the body with energy and rid it of diseases.

Some proteins act as catalysts. They accelerate chemical processes required by the body without altering. These proteins are called enzymes. These are proteins acting as regulators of the delicate chemical part of the body. It is defined as delicate because these enzymes are easily broken down and, if neutralized even slightly, can cause disease or even death.

The most significant enzymes are those that catalyze the hydrolytic reactions (those absorbing water) in the body. These are called hydrolytic or, more specifically, proteolytic enzymes.

Each group has certain simplifying duties to transport the elements introduced to the body, reducing them and making them capable of rebuilding healthy amino acid proteins.

Each hydrolytic enzyme belongs to its group in accordance with one of three functions. Those that break down carbohydrates (starch and sugar) are called amylases, those that break down fats are called lipases, and those that break down protein enzymes are called proteases. The fact that two of these three groups are found in Aloe gel explains why it is effective in the digestive process.

There are also groups of enzymes that affect other levels of functions: oxydating enzymes that break down basic elements (water, hydrogen peroxide, etc.), hydrolytic enzymes that break down solid foods, and co-enzymes that act as the basis on which compound amino acids are rebuilt.

Proper functioning of these enzymes helps the body convert fat and starch into essential proteins to provide strength and health, or to break down proteins and fats into starch to use as energy.

When all organic functions work in harmony and the enzymes and amino acids work to rebuild proteins, the body remains healthy. Even in the event of trauma or slight illness, such as stress and minimum damage, the proteolytic enzymatic process is enough to eliminate bacteria and allow the body to heal. This process is often facilitated by being integrated with vitamins and mineral salts and eating healthy foods.

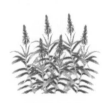

When there is serious trauma and bacteria cause damage to tissues, reducing the capacity of proteins to produce antibodies that eliminate them, the human body requires outside help. Food taken normally cannot be hydrolyzed rapidly and the body requires medication.

In most cases, this medication is found in antibiotics, most of which are highly toxic. Although they can help antibodies fight the bacteria causing the disease, they often have undesirable secondary effects, damaging other parts of the body, which becomes vulnerable to other forms of disease, and can cause allergic reactions with serious complications. This chemical ping-pong game can often cause negative results, with disease lingering until the person dies or becomes chronically ill.

Based on the certainty that the body is able to heal from within, the phytochemical message will take this direction if the appropriate signals are sent. And what if, by chance, there were a botanic element that provides the perfect complement to the biological requirements of the human body, a plant that provides all the elements the body needs to remain healthy? And what if this plant were to contain all the vitamins and mineral salts, all the sugar reducers (monosaccharides and polysaccharides) and proteolytic enzymes required to send those healing messages?

Allow me to stress that these elements that heal and revitalize tissues cannot be measured individually, but are delivered to the parts in need by the incredible penetration power of lignin and proteolytic enzyme activity. The proteolytic enzymes use the powers of the anthraquinones and detergent agents in their infinite capacity to combine and recombine, working with the nutritional elements of the plant (vitamins and mineral salts catalyzed through hydrolysis) to revitalize the protein system.

Think of the elements found in Aloe. Then think of the elementary needs of the human body. Add factor x of Aloe, capable of penetrating tissues. The presence of lignin and proteolytic enzymes enhance the plant's capacity to penetrate, which cannot be explained in laboratory tests and which we will perhaps never be able to explain. We must try to understand the true meaning of synergism, as it is here that the secret of Aloe lies and not in the study of each individual element.

In a wider perspective, credit has been given to the true healing capacity of the Aloe gel according to the individual qualities of mucopolysaccharides, proteolytic enzyme activity and amino acids. From a more limited perspective, researchers have attempted to mock this by asserting that bricks and beams are required to make a building. They asked which of these is more important. The answer is that they are all important, but only when combined.

We now at last have some knowledge of the chemical composition of Aloe, both of the gel and the entire leaf.

We know that it has various anthraquinone components, the secrets of which indicate its capacity to eliminate diseases, which have greater power of destruction than the bactericidal powers of antibiotics. Moreover, Aloe is known to have analgesic power and the ability to combat infections. It contains vitamins and mineral salts that act as nutritional elements and as agents capable of activating other curative components, all acting in synergy, to supply a natural, vegetable-based component for the biological requirements of the human body.

Great credit has been given to the idea that the elements aimed at reinforcing healing where the body requires them are due to the great penetration powers of lignin and the high level of activity of the proteolytic enzymes. Thanks to the mucopolysaccharides of Aloe and their enzymatic activity, not only do we have considerable power to penetrate and regenerate dead tissue, but also a strong structure on which healthy tissue is rebuilt by the amino acid compound.

Indications can be found in toxicological tests to reinforce my certainty that Aloe has no side effects on the human body. Moreover, hundreds of medical cards concerning thousands of cases provide further evidence that applications in situ are not toxic.

This is how **Silent Healer** concludes almost 30 pages of its authoritative study of the chemical composition of Aloe, which we have condensed to a third. It is on the basis of this important book that we begin to believe that, when it is applied, this simple recipe can offer new hope to millions of people in the world. The efficacy of the preparation is confirmed by thousands of concrete cases of healing.

Is more scientific proof required? If a fact is repeated time and again, must it be subjected to laboratory tests to verify its reliability? Do I need laboratory proof to know that if I throw a stone into the air it will fall back down?

> If you are being treated with medicines prescribed by your doctor or are to have radiotherapy, cobalt therapy, chemotherapy or other similar treatments, this does not mean you cannot use Aloe simultaneously. On the contrary, I would say that Aloe cleanses the body, eliminating the toxins and side effects caused by this type of treatment.

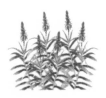

Is Aloe Toxic?

All my life I have heard people say that Aloe is toxic. After having consulted the vast amount of documentation available, including encyclopedias, I found that Aloe is believed to be toxic. I allowed this erroneous information to influence me, especially when transmitting the recipe, for fear that if someone were to exaggerate and use more Aloe than necessary, this might poison them. Being involved by chance in this subject, I have decided to clarify the matter and put an end to these rumors once and for all.

To reassure the reader on the use of this plant from the lilaceum family, I again refer to the extensive knowledge of two previously cited American works to prove that the claim Aloe is toxic is stated by people with ill intentions or who have been badly informed. We shall see through the conclusions of **Silent Healer** and **Aloe – Myth Magic Medicine** that, if someone wished to poison himself, rather than taking the prescribed amount, he would have to take masses of Aloe; in this way, even water becomes toxic. To reach the conclusion, it can be said that the degree of toxicity of Aloe is so insignificant that laboratory tests performed in the United States found measurable levels of toxicity of the plant to be almost imperceptible. Therefore, there is nothing extraordinary in the fact that in Mexico, savila – as Aloe is called by Spanish-speaking people – is used as salad, making it as toxic as lettuce! In Venezuela, it is

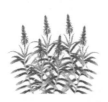

taken at breakfast, eaten in spoonfuls with a few drops of honey if too bitter.

You now know that the degree of toxicity of Aloe is minimal. If you wish to go into this subject in more depth, read the paragraphs below, obtained by studying the works cited above. If you don't have time, you can skip these pages. It is important that you rest assured when picking leaves from the plant. Believe me, it is as harmless as lettuce.

In the chapter *A Chemical Question* of the book **Silent Healer**, Aloe is analyzed. Page 75, when talking about the anthraquinone compound of the plant, states: "Anthraquinones are traditionally used as laxatives, although there are many schools of thought that attribute hidden powers to them. In a certain sense they have mysterious ingredients. Known as formidable disease exterminators, we learn that D'Amico, Benigni and others in the 1950s discovered in anthraquinones valid bactericidal agents, on the same level as antibiotics, although less toxic and more effective against viruses. This fact had been discovered previously by Lorenzetti and later confirmed by Sims and Zimmermann. We had already learned that many anthraquinones have measurable individual levels of toxicity. Nonetheless, in the sublime chemistry of Aloe vera or barbadensis, it can be seen that they are not toxic."

On page 77 of the chapter *Chrysophanic Acid* (chrysarobin), it is stated that methylanthraquinone, derived from Aloe-emodin, is known for its efficacy in the treatment of chronic skin diseases such as psoriasis and trichophytosis (a fungal skin infection).

Isolated, these have high levels of toxicity. In the case of Aloe vera, no toxicity is measured.

On page 89, under the title *Toxicology*, it says that: "We already know that certain anthraquinones found in Aloe vera gel, such as Emodin and Chrysophanic acid, have measurable levels of toxicity when observed in separate circumstances. In some cases, there is even proof that Aloe vera gel or stabilized American Aloe vera lotion and cream, which in the new formulations are now called Aloe Activator, Aloe Lotion and Aloe Vera Jelly, measured respectively, have no level of toxicity. This is more important than it seems at first sight, once the toxic levels of all things belonging to the animal kingdom are measured. In toxicological experiments known as LD-50s, some animals (dogs, rabbits, mice and monkeys) were exposed to rays called death rays, meaning they were selected to receive levels of exposure capable of killing them. In the case of topical applications, they were exposed to acute doses of rays at levels high enough to produce lethal irritations. The list of cases proving that Aloe vera is not toxic is considerably extensive.

I will divide the study into three parts to prove my point of view. One part was performed in the Lakeland Laboratories, sponsored by Aloe Vera of America Inc.; the other two were conducted by independent research groups with no possibility of interaction. All three cases gave results confirming this.

With regard to the first example, a study had already been performed in 1986 by Sam Houston, in the Brooke General

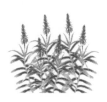

Hospital in Texas, and by the Baylor Faculty of Dentology in Dallas.

In this study, Dr. E.R. Zimmermann, D.D.S., pathology head of the Baylor Faculty, Dr. James Brasher and Dr. C.K. Collins observed the effects on the extract of fibroblasts from rabbit kidneys, sensitized by irritants. At this point it is important to stress that rabbit tissues, in many ways similar to those of humans, have the further advantage of being thirteen times more susceptible to toxicity than human tissue.

In the tests by Brasher and Zimmermann, Aloe vera was tested against indomethacin, a non-steroid drug, and prednisolone, a potent cortico-steroid.

Like Aloe vera, indomethacin was purported to possess strong analgesic and antipruritic properties. Prednisolone, like Aloe vera, was an acknowledged anti-inflammatory agent. Owing to this common anti-inflammatory property, it was decided to compare them. Tests were carried out on two levels. First, the three were tested on the rabbit tissue culture He la Cells for their ability to stimulate cell division and promote healing. In a 72-hour period, Aloe vera had far outstripped both the prednisolone and the indomethacin in this tissue-growing ability. Furthermore, under an electronic microscopic amplification of 500,000/1, the Brasher/Zimmermann group was able to observe an accelerated yet normal growth of tissue, one with no trace of carcinoma.

More important for our purposes, the Aloe gel exhibited negligible levels of toxicity in its cell tissue, while the prednisolone and indomethacin levels were much higher. The gel supplied was the one developed by Aloe Vera of America Inc.

These tests confirmed the conclusions reached by Lakeland Laboratories in 1966. In the experiments performed on a large number of rabbits, pathologists Henry Cobble and Dr. Mertin Grossman found no toxicity in any of the vital organs or in the muscle tissue or skin of the rabbits. Some of the animals that had ingested doses of Aloe vera lost weight, but this was attributed to normal lack of nutritional elements in the diet. Toxicity was insignificant, even at extremely high doses (over 20 g per kilo). In 1968, these experiments were repeated on a large scale in the Hazelton Laboratories in Falls Church, Virginia. Under the direction of pathologist William M. Busey, M.D., the experiments with ID50 were conducted on laboratory animals, with large oral doses given to the mice and eight dogs, and large dermal doses applied to the group of white mice.

All these animals were exposed to extremely high doses for a period of 14 days. Once again, the results were excellent. Dr. Busey's assessments were as follows: The mice were observed as regards incidence of mortality and toxic effects after 14 days. The large oral dose of LD50 given exceeded 2.15 g/kg (extremely high).

"Single oral doses of the stabilized Aloe vera gel were administered by stomach tube to four groups of mongrel dogs, one male and one female in each group. There were no deaths 14 days after the dose; therefore, the oral dose tolerated by the dogs could exceed 31.6 g/kg of their body weight.

"The stabilized Aloe vera gel was also analyzed in cases of dermal irradiation and for its toxicity over a period of 24 hours of application to the abdomen (with the skin scraped) of the white mice. No deaths occurred. The large dose of LD50 was therefore above 10g/kg of body weight. There were minimum dermal irritations."

There is also convincing research on the curative capabilities in the form of bacteriologic records and stories of recent medical cases.

The last reference from **Silent Healer** regarding the toxicity of Aloe is taken from page 92 under the heading *Abstract*: "From our toxicological records, we affirm that Aloe vera has no side effects on the human body. Moreover hundreds of medical records, taken from thousands of cases once again confirm the lack of toxicity in local applications."

By reading the second work cited (**Aloe – Myth Magic Medicine**, by Odus M. Hennessee and Bill R. Cook), we find new affirmations on the subject. On page 11, there is a summary of the characteristics of the plant. It is worthwhile drawing attention to the content of the skin of Aloe: "Scientific studies have proved that the most efficacious use of Aloe comes from a balanced mixture of these three elements. The gel plays its role when mixed adequately with the juice, but is of little value on its own.

"The sap contains most of the medicinal agents and is much more than a laxative or treatment for minor skin ailments. Some are convinced that the outermost skin has no curative virtues, notwithstanding the fact it contains a large number of nutritional elements, found in the sap and gel. Previous studies have proved that the skin is neither harmful nor dangerous, as many people have claimed. Logic suggests that use of the whole leaf is preferable."

We find fervent defense of the therapeutic qualities of the plant in a long citation on page 56. "Notwithstanding the use of the sap as healing agent in ancient recipes, almost all promulgators stated that not only did the sap cause allergic reactions but was also dangerous and that, consequently, it could not be used in products with Aloe vera. In order to sell their products they created the myth that only the gel was the chosen agent, supporting this idea by spreading the word, which did not correspond to the truth, that modern studies had proved that the sap was toxic for human tissue and that it caused allergic reactions. In complete contrast to this assertion, all studies published on toxicity instead prove that the toxic effect of Aloe is inexistent or almost so and that it does not cause allergies. Perhaps the promulgators are somewhat confused as they only have a superficial knowledge of the chemistry of Aloe. To cite just one example of this possible lack of true knowledge, it must be borne in mind that the sap is scientifically recognized as a glucose anthraquinone. According to the Merck index, an anthraquinone is a synthetic substance used to produce tinctures, which have generalized toxicity and which can cause skin irritations or cutaneous rashes.

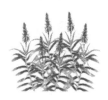

"Therefore incomplete information without terms for comparison, based on this definition of synthetic anthraquinones, may lead to the erroneous conclusion that the sap coincidentally still used as a tincture is toxic, causes cutaneous rashes or allergic reactions. Perhaps another source of this idea that the plant is toxic or poisonous comes from the Russian Encyclopedia, which states that a certain species of Aloe that grows in Russia is apparently poisonous. Nonetheless, this species has no relation with Aloe vera. We could continue to cite various cases of erroneous convictions concerning Aloe vera, which have been repeated endlessly by badly informed people. Often these specific convictions are related to the source of these ideas. Further descriptions merely report the original error, without bothering to prove the validity of their source. This has led to an increase in confusion."

On page 59, it states that the curative powers are found in the whole plant and not in one of its isolated elements: "Many researches have proposed a possible relation of synergism between all the substances contained in Aloe vera. Synergism means the capacity of all the physical and chemical components of the plant to function together, in order to bring greater benefit than the benefit given by the single elements individually. If this theory is correct, it would explain the fact that Aloe is not toxic and does not have allergic effects although it contains agents that, isolated or alone, can cause toxic and allergic effects."

On page 61, it is explained that Aloe acts without causing damage as its components are wisely distributed: "After having seen the results of this research (performed in the Burns Centre of the University of Chicago, 1982), it can be assumed that Aloe vera functions without causing toxic or allergic effects, as its nutritional elements and the water it contains act as a buffer.

"The nutritional elements are also necessary for the growth and function of the tissue. The plant controls (or eliminates) infections by means of its natural antiseptic agents – sulphur, phenols, lupeol, salicylic acid, cinnamic acid and nitrogenised urea. It controls inflammation with its anti-inflammatory fatty acids, which are cholesterol, campesterol, Beta-sitosterol. It limits or alleviates pain thanks to its content of lupeol, salicylic acid and magnesium. By acting together these elements and the other components of the leaves cause this synergetic relationship. This provides us with a reasonable explanation for the numerous reports concerning the fact that Aloe eliminates many internal and external infections and reduces pain efficaciously. Chemistry explains Aloe's capacity to act as efficacious treatment for burns, cuts and abrasions, and in the treatment of inflammatory diseases such as rheumatic fever, arthritis of all types, diseases of the skin, mouth, esophagus, stomach, intestine, colon and other internal organs such as the kidneys, spleen, pancreas and liver. It is important to remember that the anti-inflammatory and anti-bacterial agents are found in the sap and skin of the plant and not in the gel. At the same time it must be borne in mind that the fundamental nutritional elements and other agents are widely distributed throughout the plant – sap, gel and skin – and about 98% of the water is in the gel. This knowledge would help to put an end to the pseudo-scientific rumors, especially to the conviction that the gel of the plant is solely responsible for the curative capacities of Aloe vera. The gel is important as a buffer agent. Therefore, the theory of a synergetic relationship is backed both by Science and History.

"In my search for the truth, I have a chemical explanation for Aloe vera's capacity to heal, control or eliminate a great number of diseases caused by microbes, to calm or eliminate pain and to control inflammation. We know, as it has been confirmed repeatedly, that the plant has all these capacities and many more besides. Nonetheless, we shall not as yet discuss Aloe's ability to eliminate water from tissue, to aid digestion, to balance acidity in the body, to eliminate or visibly reduce scars, to regenerate piliferous follicles, to renew damaged skin, to restore healthy skin color and to offer many other benefits, to be explored as soon as we pass from theory to practice."

On page 65, chapter 9, the specific subject is *Toxicology*. Perhaps it would be useful to copy it ipsis litteris, but it is rather long, so I have tried to summarize it. It starts by saying: "In the work **O superfaturamento do Aloe Vera**, F.D.A. presents an unsolved problem in which the author of the article claims that the juice of Aloe vera can be toxic if swallowed. At the same time, the author states that, in a study performed in 1974, it was proved that the juice of Aloe vera was not toxic for mice. In fact, after having carefully studied the literature concerning the possible toxicity of Aloe vera, he proved that Aloe vera is not only non-toxic, but it truly helps to regenerate tissue. In 1959, the same F.D.A. oddly concluded that Aloe vera was not toxic. Or at least this is the impression given by Gunnar Gjerstad and T.D. Riner in the article *Current state of Aloe as a panacea.* Gjerstad and Finer reviewed data by E.P. Pendergrass concerning the efficiency of Aloe vera in treating burns from X-rays and other forms of radiation, and admitted that the Aloe ointment used by Pendergrass regenerated the skin tissue.

"The following part of the chapter proposes to answer the question: Is Aloe vera toxic? Does it cause necrosis or regenerate tissue? Although it is totally clear that Aloe vera heals and regenerates tissue, the doubt persists in those requiring further proof of positive results. In other words, the skeptics want other specific studies proving that Aloe is not harmful to tissue and regenerates it. This study was published by Hazleton Laboratories Inc., a subsidiary of TRW, from Falls Church, V.A., in January 1969. The toxicity index was observed in the work *Dermal applications on rabbits for 13 days with stabilized Aloe Vera Gel - Final Report.* The Hazleton researchers concluded that repeated applications of Aloe vera caused no histopathologic change in any of the tissues examined nor in the liver, kidneys or skin of the white rabbits." Let us examine the article by R. R. Zimmermann, 1969: Effects of prednisolone, indomethacin and Aloe Vera Gel on tissue culture cells, at the Federal Dental Services. After having used Aloe vera gel in various concentrations, Zimmermann determined that it was less toxic than prednisolone or indomethacin when tested in Grey type He La cells and in rabbit kidney fibroblasts. It is important to observe that this study concluded that with Aloe vera the cells studied lived for two thirds longer than normal expectations.

"Therefore, Aloe vera does not merely not kill the cells, but it stimulates them to live in a healthy condition for a long period."

To conclude the subject of toxicity in Aloe, we refer to what one dentist practices in his profession. Check this out on page 84: Dr. Wolfe recommends that this gel be applied around permanent crowns and along the edges of the gum around these crowns with a light massage. With regard to periodontal studies, Dr. Wolfe states: "In gingivitis with acute ulcerative necrosis, the objective is to eliminate the symptoms, so that complete cleansing can be performed. Usually the first visit consists in removing tartar. After oral hygiene the patient is advised to apply Aloe vera as often as possible to the parts involved with an interdental stimulator or irrigation syringe. For endodontic use, Dr. Wolfe stated that Aloe vera is efficacious as a channel lubricator. Before injecting into the channel, he says, he injects a small amount of Aloe vera into the file for cleaning the channels, without worrying if a little gel passes the apex, as research has proved that Aloe vera is not toxic and regenerates cell tissue."

It would be ideal to report the content of both books, as together they form an encyclopedia on Aloe. To conclude this chapter, I have chosen some of the most practical passages.

1. "It is believed that the Aloe vera plant has no curative virtues until its leaves grow large (over one pound, 454 g) and are from two to four years old. However, this idea is disproved

by the fact that even plants with small leaves (3 or 4 ounces, about 70 g) grown on the window sill at home give extraordinary benefits.

"A shoot that grows from the root of the mother plant starts to produce sap in a few weeks; this is why pets, especially cats, eat the shoots as soon as they appear. It is not the age of the plant that makes it more efficacious, although the larger leaves are more important for the success of the commercial producer." It can be deduced that even the young leaf is useful, as it already contains the properties of the plant.

2. "For example, the Ebbers Papyrus states that Aloe was used as a beauty product by men and women alike, internally and externally, to make their health and beauty stand out, inside and out. Beauty products in ancient times were the expression of the idea that health and beauty went hand in hand." Health and beauty are gifts that could be sought by persistent men and women.

3. "Only after reading something about Aloe vera and having tested it in 1973, was I able to find respite from my skin problems, using an Aloe-based jelly product, which was a combination of sap and gel. Unfortunately, at that time I didn't know that Aloe could be used internally; I accepted the erroneous general belief that the sap was poisonous. I started to take 100% high quality Aloe vera just six years ago, after starting to seriously study the historical and scientific findings concerning the plant. I knew Aloe was a genuine product, as I had prepared it myself. To my surprise and delight my allergies

disappeared completely immediately after I started to take it regularly.

"I found that if I didn't take it regularly my allergies returned, so I started to experiment. Between January and June 1984 I took Aloe for regular periods of two weeks. I discovered that when I took the product every day, my allergies disappeared and when I stopped taking it, they came back. Although I hadn't completed my research to find out why Aloe worked, I benefited personally from it and, as I didn't want my allergies to return, I started to take Aloe every day, and still continue to do so. Today I know I have no allergies, but I also know through experience that if I stop taking Aloe the symptoms return. Above all, my chronic topical dermatitis has completely disappeared. However, Aloe does much more than curing my allergies. By taking it every day I have completely eliminated chronic indigestion, which caused constipation and kidney infections. I am now completely cleared of hemorrhoids and I believe this is due to systematically applying the Aloe ointment and also because my digestion and bowels function more regularly. My cholesterol level has decreased by half, even if I believe this is due to changes in diet. I was able to ascertain that taking Aloe attenuates pain and the advance of arthritis in my knees and ankles, caused by contusions due to accidents I had when I played sports and for which I had to have four important operations (in my younger days). It is true that the pains in my legs have disappeared without returning since I started to take Aloe every day. Aloe has increased my energy and I can add that I have had no colds, flu or other types of infection for the last five years, while my friends suffer from these problems continually. I could go on but believe you already know enough."

Is more complete proof required? Aloe has given good results for all the ailments mentioned above. Another myth has been disproved: Aloe can be taken continuously, thus confirming the theory that the degree of toxicity is truly insignificant.

4. "Please pay particular attention to the fact that in the previous description we said that the Reverend Thompson was under medical surveillance during the cycle of treatment at home (after having had over 22 operations to the skin due to leg burns caused by a fuel container exploding) with Aloe ointment and that a second doctor examined him to confirm that his wounds had healed. Not treating ourselves with modern medicine may be seen an act of ignorance by us. It is without doubt beneficial to point out that the patient's body belongs to him and not to the doctor. The simple truth is that in the past patients tended to depend largely on doctors. The specialist is naturally the first person who should be consulted in the case of disease or lesions. And if after years of treatment you are still suffering or have had little or no improvement? It seems obvious that in this case the person is entitled to seek alternative methods of treatment." There is a great deal of wisdom in these lines. Another thing is to do as many Brazilians do, that is take self-medication, or go to the doctor for a simple little cold."

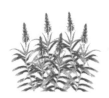

5. "I too have seen prodigious healings performed using Aloe. The most spectacular example is probably a much respected local trader, Lyle Ball.

"In February 1998, Lyle had radical treatment for skin cancer on both arms, from the elbow down to the back of the hand. He received treatment for a period of two to three weeks with chemical products to treat the burns caused by cancer. Naturally, he was in great pain after the treatment. His doctor had given him painkillers and topical ointments, but Lyle said they weren't working. His wife had heard about Aloe vera and had suggested he try it to calm the pain and help to heal the burns. After about 48 hours from the last session of chemotherapy, Lyle started to use a combination of concentrated Aloe ointment together with a concentrated Aloe gel spray. He said his main aim was to combat the pain. This decreased almost immediately after using the ointment and spray, and after a week he had no more pain. The burns on Mr. Ball's arms healed completely in 11 days (from 18th to 29th February 1988). At the time of writing, the skin on both Mr. Ball's arms and hands has healed completely and there are only a few scars." Stories like this are heard from people who use Aloe to cure their ailments.

To sum up, we can conclude by thanking God for this wonderful plant He gave to nature, at the disposal of the poor, but also of the most powerful, when through arrogance and stubbornness they are not totally small-minded about topics such as these. Perhaps God will be generous and open their minds.

So why is it stated in some encyclopedias that Aloe is toxic? According to phytology technician Dr. Aldo Facetti, it is the concentrate of Aloe that is toxic. To obtain this, it would be necessary to infuse or distill from 30 to 50 plants, including the roots. However, in its natural state, Aloe is as harmless as lettuce. This information disproves the theory that Aloe causes abortion; likewise, there is no danger in using it to cure hemorrhoids. (I can assure you that Aloe cures hemorrhoids!). If you wish to be certain and rest assured, use the plant in its natural state; in this state, it is harmless. Use it always, both for internal health problems and external injuries.

If you fear that you could be allergic to Aloe (extremely rare!) you can test it on yourself at home. Cut two centimeters of Aloe leaf and apply it to the skin behind the ear or the armpit for about two minutes. If the skin on which the Aloe is applied becomes itchy or inflamed, you are allergic both to natural Aloe and other commercially produced products. However, I repeat this is extremely rare.

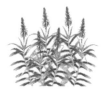

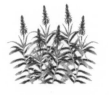

Aloe and AIDS

Studies performed ten years ago by Bill McAnalley show that another carrisyn polysaccharide has been isolated. A Canadian study identified it as Acemannan, suitable for antiviral activity. The substance was patented by Carrington Laboratories. There is clinical proof showing its efficacy to stimulate the immune system in patients suffering from AIDS, preventing expansion of the HIV virus. We shall discuss these findings together with the reader.

When I returned to Europe from the Middle East in August 1995, I came across **Silent Healer, a modern study on Aloe Vera** by Bill C. Coats, R.Ph, with Robert Ahola, in a special translation sponsored by Toho Cosmetic, and **Aloe – Myth Magic Medicine: Aloe Vera Across Time**, by Odus M. Hennessee and Bill R. Cook, the most complete studies I had read to date on Aloe used on people and animals, over 20 years of experience by the authors. It seems incredible, but I felt at home when reading these books, as I had also had a similar experience, mutatis mutandis, especially with people rather than animals.

With specific reference to AIDS, on pages 88-91 of the book **Aloe – Myth Magic Medicine**, we find the text "AIDS – a new frontier in research," pages 88-91. Because of its importance and clarity, we shall cite the entire passage. It proves that, unknown to us, Aloe was already being used by people with AIDS in the

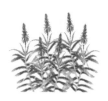

United States and with the same effects obtained by us. Here is the text:

Since 1987, it is commonplace to hear from those with AIDS from the Dallas-Fort Worth area, that Aloe juice or a drug (polymannoacetate) deriving from it provided equal relief from the symptoms of the disease and had protected those with the virus, with none of the symptoms of AIDS that cause the disease to advance.

The work was performed at the Dallas-Fort Worth Medical Centre, Grand Prairie, Texas and is considered important, owing to the status of the doctors involved; it would be an act of negligence not to report the results obtained to date.

It is extremely important to understand that this research does not show that Aloe vera cures AIDS. Instead, it shows that excellent results were obtained in all cases examined. In most of the tests, Aloe vera prevented the disease from advancing. In other words, Aloe vera does not cure AIDS but is an extremely efficacious treatment.

This was presented for the first time in an article: *The Aloe drug can replace AZT without danger of toxicity*, in the **Medical World News**, December 1987 edition. The article refers to research work by Dr. H.R. McDaniel, according to whom, a substance contained in the Aloe plant forecasts the possibility of reinforcing the immune system in AIDS patients and preventing human immune deficiency virus from advancing without any toxic side effects.

The results of Dr. McDaniel's study showed that the symptoms of seventeen AIDS sufferers decreased substantially when they were given 1,000 mg per day of the drug for a duration of three months. After this period, the symptoms of six patients in the advanced stage of the disease had improved by 20% while less seriously ill patients obtained an improvement averaging around 71%. Dr. McDaniel also reported the results of his research in the combined meeting with the American Society of Clinical Pathologists and the College of American Pathologists.

He says that: "Fever and night sweats, diarrhea and general infections were eliminated and there were significant improvements in all patients, with a corresponding decrease in the cultures of HIV positive cells and a decrease in the levels of the principal antigen of HIV."

The erythrocyte mass increased in all but one patient, and in twelve who were initially leucopoenic, there had been a slight increase in the white cell count after treatment.

No toxic effects were observed in twenty-nine patients who received the experimental drug.

It is therefore clear that high quality Aloe juice can ease AIDS symptoms. This does not surprise us, as the drug (polymannoacetate) is produced from the plant and must be found in the juice.

An article by Irwin Frank, published on July 12, 1988 in the **Dallas Times Herald**, quotes Dr. Terry Pulse as saying that "580 g (20 ounces) of Aloe vera juice with the drug stabilized in the Aloe, were administered orally to 69 AIDS patients." (Dr. Irwin apparently means the juice of stabilized Aloe vera.)

According to the article, Pulse states that the patients treated with the drug were classified as those who "would never have improved or recovered," but by following the treatment they would be able to "go back to their normal work." The article quoted the words of Pulse according to whom "these patients recovered their energy, as the symptoms had almost totally disappeared – and this was the case in 81% of the patients who took the drug."

He adds that the patients with AIDS who showed no symptoms of the disease continued not to show any while taking the drug deriving from Aloe vera.

Pulse states that "the earlier a patient takes the drug, the sooner he will recover." His patients took 580 g (20 ounces) of the liquid each day, "and I kept them alive in this way for a long time, some for over two years."

"We have had deaths," he continues, "but the death of these patients can be attributed to chemotherapy for skin

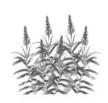

or other cancers, or to taking combinations of other drugs that paralyzed their immune system, such as AZT."

When we asked the significance of his studies and his therapy to treat or cure AIDS, Pulse answered: "They show that, until there is a magic bullet, this solution is temporary and prolongs the life (of AIDS patients) at a much lower cost than AZT."

After having read this article, we were able to obtain copies of the actual research data published by Dr. Pulse, together with his collaborators, H.R. McDaniel and T. Reg. Watson, all from the Dallas-Fort Worth Medical Centre.

The information given by Pulse was checked to eliminate confusion concerning what had actually been used in the study, whether the product was Aloe vera juice or a drug, or both, and in what percentage.

From this data and further investigation, it seems that Aloe vera juice, in its natural state, is just as efficacious in treating AIDS as the cold stabilized drug obtained from it. Naturally, anyone with AIDS who considers Aloe vera efficacious in the treatment of their condition should be extremely cautious when purchasing juice with 100% of Aloe vera and, as we have often said, check that it is nothing but water. We repeat that true Aloe is amber in color and tastes bitter.

You can imagine my surprise on reading this article! In other words, it confirmed what I had been practicing for years. This article gave me great confidence regarding what I had, to date, practiced as a layman, without the support of the experience of others, motivated merely by the will to help those suffering.

I had helped AIDS sufferers almost by chance, as people involved in this problem who had heard of cases of cancer healings, called me. "If Aloe has had good results with cancer," they said, "perhaps it could be of help in treating AIDS!" I myself reasoned in a different way: "If Aloe can cure tumors, why not AIDS?" Below I have described some cases of people who sought my help.

Using the same recipe proposed in this book, I helped a twenty-year-old Muslim from Ramallah near Jerusalem. Again, I only used Aloe in its natural state, picked from the plant and prepared without performing any stabilization process which, in any case, I did not even know.

I must mention that the first time the boy came to me in a wheelchair in a terrible state, accompanied by his family. The second time he came alone, on his own two feet. The joy his family showed when they saw me again was immense: they asked for my permission to pray to Allah, there and then, facing Mecca and kneeling reverently, according to Islamic custom. I wonder what became of Alex and whether he is still alive.

After taking three jars of the preparation, an AIDS patient, Vincenzo M. from Lascari, Palermo Italy, was employed as a nurse in a hospital in Palermo. If the virus had not been halted, no chief consultant in his right mind would have employed someone with the HIV virus as a nurse, a person who assists sick people and is in constant danger of transmitting the disease. I saw Vincenzo in Palermo in 1995 at his work. He looked just like any other young man of his age. At first sight, no one could imagine that he had AIDS.

Eagle, from Cagliari, Sardinia in Italy, who had AIDS, kept in contact over the phone with Bethlehem and received the necessary instructions. After three or four jars of the preparation, she had tests in Turin, where Dr. Maurizio Grandi turned her inside out, examining her thoroughly. The first tests showed counts of around 500. In the second tests, they had risen to around 700. Naturally, Eagle continued taking the potion. When I visited the island in mid-June, I met her personally.

She is a very attractive girl, strong and with a healthy glow on her cheeks. No one would ever imagine she has AIDS. She told me that the counts had reached 1000, a number considered reasonable, within the norm. Good God, how vibrant she was! What a will to live, joyful over her victory to this point!

Perhaps the most spectacular case concerning AIDS is the one of Dr. Cristina Sannia from Cagliari, Sardinia in Italy. After work, this doctor of Greek-Orthodox origin takes her Jeep and drives around the island looking for Aloe, which grows abundantly in the region. She uses it to treat almost three thousand people with AIDS on the island. She does this of her own free will. Owing to this, she took part in a conference in the Sinnai Council amphitheatre in Cagliari. There the doctor spoke of the excellent results obtained with her patients, thanks to my recipe. She said that usually, after having taken three jarfuls, patients went back to a normal life. With a stomach that is working well, better appetite, healthy skin color and liver in good condition, the patients often return to all their former activities.

Two months after I returned to my own country, after a series of interviews with the mass media, starting with an interview at Radio Guaiba on September 2, 1995 (conducted by doctor and journalist Dr. Abraao Wiriogron, in his traditional program Medicine and Health, with a large audience and with the participation of Dr. Sergio Reutmann), I started to record a long list of telephone calls, about twenty, mainly from Porto Alegre, informing me of the health of people with the AIDS virus: improved general health, better appetite, the strength to walk, healthy glow on their cheeks, etc. In a word, after two or three doses, there was considerable improvement.

To conclude this chapter, I wish to stress that people should not deceive themselves! Aloe neither cures nor eliminates the HIV virus. It merely prevents it from advancing, which is important in view of the seriousness of the disease. In the case of cancer, Aloe is undoubtedly a cure, renewing all the affected cells, truly regenerating the weakened immune system, discussed in a separate chapter of this book. Unfortunately, this is not the case with AIDS: Aloe does not cure AIDS. In any case, we are pleased to state that there is a way of offering a better quality of life to AIDS sufferers for the rest of their lives, although the best thing would be to eliminate the virus completely. We hope that medicine and science together find this cure as soon as possible, as the forecasts for the coming years are disastrous, a general tragedy unless the solution is found soon.

As can be observed in the article quoted above, Aloe acts positively on the HIV virus, without any negative side effects, such as those caused by AZT and other drugs. Aloe is accessible to all, even those who are poor. Research performed by Harvard University in the United States in 1993 raised the question of whether the benefits of AZT in the anti-AIDS therapy were cancelled out by side effects such as anemia, nausea, vomiting and tiredness. In 1995, another medicine called Indinavir, or MK-639, managed to reduce the quantity of virus present in the body by up to 99% and increased the number of CD-4, one of the cell types that defends the body, 50 times.

As these drugs are only accessible to the privileged classes of society, the poorer can but make use of Aloe, which responds well and has two advantages: there are no negative side effects and it is available to all.

The same can be said of the cocktail of medicines recently mentioned in the press. Over and above its side effects, it costs 1,200 US dollars per month for each patient. The Aloe recipe costs less than $100 for a 16 oz. bottle.

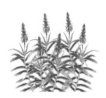

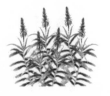

Face to Face

Monologue by Father Romano Zago to the Aloe Leaf – Almost a Prayer

Each time I prepare a jar of the Aloe, honey and distillate preparation, I go to the plant alone, humbly. Slowly, with the same respect as someone looking at a rare object, an animal in extinction or a work of art.

I go to the plant with a sharp knife, not with the intent of attacking her, not as a superior being or her possessor, but as a creature on equal grounds as concerns condition and level.

I stand before the plant as an incomplete and impotent being in the hope and confidence that she can help me to solve a predicament. I greet her as I would greet a person:

"Hello, beautiful creature! I am not here to hurt you. On the contrary, as I know you are beneficial, I ask you to give me what our Creator gave you. I need it. All that God created is good. You are the essence of God, perfect, beautiful, harmonious. God has deposited rich substances within you. I wish to take advantage of these. If I do not take them, they will never be used for their purpose. Just as all living beings, you were born and grew, but will die, returning to the dust in the ground that produced you. But if I pick you, you will offer all your substances and give everything good you know. So, let me pick you as I

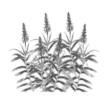

would a beautiful rose. Only you know the wonders you possess internally and feel the ecstasy of fertility."

When I take the leaf gently in my hand, I caress it from top to bottom, passing the serrated edge of the spines over the palm of my hand as if to make her understand that she is not ferocious and aggressive and I whisper:

"You will suffer a little but I know no other way of taking you so that you can do the job for which you were created. Come with me, come! I have chosen you because I know you are willing to put what you know into practice. Consider yourself fortunate. Yes, your companions will remain for future use should they be needed; if not, they will die and their lives will have been futile. Just as a flower that blooms in the middle of the Amazon forest or a wave in the middle of the ocean, without being able to exploit their potential fully.

"I will cut some leaves near the stem with a sharp cut, so that you lose none of your essence, none of your extraordinary and healing sap."

With a gentle cut of the blade I remove the leaf from the stem to which it is attached, without tearing, crushing or shaking it.

After having cleaned off dust and removed the spines, it is combined with genuine honey to the distillate chosen and blended well.

While the three elements are being mixed and blended, I place my hands over the bowl of the blender like a lid, as if to transmit all my energy to the preparation. When it is ready, I address the plant for the last time to ask her to perform her mission using the vital force within her.

"Now go and do what you have to. In a body created by God there must be no disease, pain, discord or unbalance. Free the body entrusted to you from disease, by doing what you know how to do.

"I love you. Yes, it is true that I chose you from many others of the same type. Take advantage of this opportunity and perform the mission that the Lord planned when He created you. It is now time for ecstasy. I know that as soon as your mission has been performed you will thank me for the opportunity you have been given. I too am extremely grateful to you for the help you will give to that sick body. I want to apologize and thank you for this service that you have been called to provide, with great love. Go and do what you know how to do."

"Blessed is the Lord who with Aloe and all nature, has given us many chances to cure our diseases. Once healed, live with joy a new life of thanks and praise. Let us be allowed to discover and use all resources for our good and spend our lives in continual act of grace! Amen."

Father Romano Zago, OFM

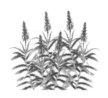

If you suffer from diabetes or suspect that the honey is not organic and could therefore upset you, prepare the blend required for that day each day. Use fruit, grains or vegetables in place of honey. Some people are allergic to honey. In this case, if you are allergic to honey, you may become constipated. This can be avoided by replacing honey with freshly squeezed juice.

If honey is genuine, it does not harm a diabetic. There is even a recipe for treating diabetes: one spoonful of honey, at least ten years old, first thing in the morning on an empty stomach.

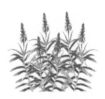

Parting Comments

On these modest pages, you have read the story of the trajectory of a recipe, as if it were a meteorite; a homemade, inexpensive recipe that cures cancer.

We have indicated that preference should be given to Aloe grown at home, as commercialized products which have been subjected to stabilization processes can have reduced curative properties. Use Aloe from your own home, the same ornamental plant on the windowsill, the same used as a hair tonic or to treat small cuts or scalds from household accidents. It is the same plant: use it whenever you need. Commercial products which, owing to the greed of manufacturers are expensive, can also lose their virtues. Follow the indications given in this book. The knowledge gained is more than sufficient to help you in particular circumstances. If you are not in an area that grows Aloe arborescens, seek a reliable commercial source of the recipe.

The preparation has no contraindications. The use of Aloe is discredited because it didn't cause any reactions in vitro in the laboratory. We have experiences of in vitro reactions in Brazil and abroad. On their own, these are insignificant experiences aimed only at satisfying scientific interest. In the history of medicine, there are several cases of substances that had no reaction in vitro, but that were marketed, thanks to their reaction in nature. Therefore, not only substances tested in the

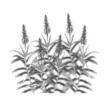

laboratory are accepted by medicine. Medicine ends up using all the experiences and facts that often, after occurring accidentally or casually, become part of the heritage of humanity.

The fact that in some cases my preparation can cause diarrhea may frighten people. In fact it does cause it; it must cause it. This is part of the expectations. The phenomenon can be explained as follows: toxins that have deposited in the body at last find a normal exit route. Another route is through urine. The third is by excretion through the pores. The fourth is through vomiting. This is all natural. It is the wisdom of the body trying to cleanse itself. When this symptom appears, so-called experts state that diarrhea causes loss of potassium. So what should we say about radiotherapy, chemotherapy, antibiotics and analgesics with their gruesome procession of negative side effects? When there is diarrhea, which seldom lasts longer than two or three days, any loss of potassium can be offset by eating a banana each day; this fruit is rich in this alkaline metal required by the body. Watch out for alarmism; it may not be true.

Love yourself. Look after your health. Do not smoke, drink or take drugs. Alcohol and smoke damage the body in arithmetical proportions, drugs in geometrical proportions. Look at the world. It is beautiful and it is also yours! However, remember that there are others living here, with the same rights and duties. Try to live your life well. Let us make the world a more beautiful and just place to live, where everyone has the chance to live. The country we live in is in a continent that contains 75%

of the specimens of flora from the planet. Let's try to explore and study it lovingly. Let's use these riches for the good of humanity. Our extensive territory could easily accommodate the entire population of China, with food and housing for all, if it weren't for the action of mediators. We must try to live in peace, in mutual respect, even for the sole fact that we are all human beings.

In truth, man must learn to love himself. How can he love others like himself if he is going towards self-destruction through drugs, smoking, alcohol, pesticides, pollution, atomic explosions?

Only after having learned to truly love himself will man be able to love his fellow man. Then we shall be near to perfection.

If you obtained any benefit from using Aloe, please write to the publishing house about the results obtained; they will forward any letters periodically to Father Romano. Your case could help to solve the problem of another human being.

Fr. Romano Zago, OFM
Caixa Postal 2330
90001-970 Porto Alegre, RS-Brazil
Email: freiromanozago@bol.com.br

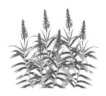

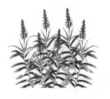

Cancer Can Be Cured Appendix

The Scientific Monographic History of Aloe Vera and Aloe Arborescens

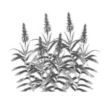

To The Readers

By Father Romano Zago, OFM

The inspiration for writing this second book that is now added as an Appendix came from my fellow Brazilian co-nationals, who allowed me to dedicate my body and soul to this project. According to recent statistics, Brazil is one of the richest natural resource countries in the world, yet its approximately 50 million people – about one third of the country's total population – continue to live in poverty.

People like the Brazilians are unable to imagine the idea of having a health plan. Public health in Brazil has been trans-formed into a professional degradation, poorly remunerated for the way the system works. This has created an extremely precarious health care system. It is not unusual to find patients waiting months for a doctor's visit. Often, they end up dying in the hospital corridors. Medicines and other aids are inaccessible because of their high cost. It is for this reason that I have decided to write this book. I would like to try and share in their pain, and I apologize for expressing my opinion regarding this matter. But it is the only way I am able to ease my conscience. I realize that my attempt is not enough, but it is what I have learned to do. If this book helps decrease suffering and contri-butes to the increase in economic possibilities for my people, then so be it. It will be a good reason to cry for joy and for my commemoration.

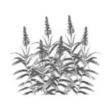

Aloe is a Food

It is important to know that, for its impressive arsenal of medicinal properties, Aloe is defined as being proudly "self-sufficient" in chemical terms, leaving the rest to economic matters. Aloe is widely known to man through ancient cultures but is often ignored by arrogant Western allopathic medicine.

If you choose to take Aloe, you will benefit nutritionally because it is a complete food. Aloe is a collection of useful and essential nutritional elements such as enzymes, vitamins, proteins, amino acids, minerals, oils, monosaccharides, polysaccharides, etc. In 1873, German medicine during the time of Bismarck had already dealt with more than 300 medicines that contained Aloe. Today's literature confirms that research being done in laboratories is honestly and objectively searching for the truth. It is peculiar that misinformed people insist that Aloe does not contain any element useful for medicinal purposes. The refusal to recognize the positive and curative effects that plants or herbal hydrotherapy have on people demonstrates a widespread ignorance about Aloe.

Science is used when one has to search for the truth. The Gospel states: "The truth will save you."

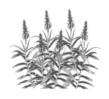

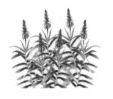

The Difference Between Aloe Vera Barbadensis Miller and Aloe Arborescens Miller

The botanical type of Aloe, already classified within the Liliacee family, is currently included within the Aloacee family. This includes a large variety of approximately 350 species of plants found throughout the entire planet, including evergreen, large and leafy plants, and those which have elongated, colorful flowers that range from orange to scarlet red. The leaves and bark of these plants come in various shapes and sizes. Their dimensions range from large-scale plants to miniature ones. The smaller ones are used mainly for food, herbal hydrotherapeutic, and cosmetic purposes. Aloe Barbadensis Miller (Aloe vera) and Aloe Arborescens Miller are included in this group and are widely known for their innate characteristics.

Aloe Barbadensis Miller (Aloe Vera)

Aloe Barbadensis Miller (Aloe vera) is a perennial plant with green succulent and full foliage. The leaves contain a vast amount of gel in their external cuticle. The various substances present in these leaves highlight an acemannan polysaccharide involved in the process of immuno-modulation and an anti-inflammatory action that is significant in the field of hydrotherapy. Aloina found in the plant belongs to the anthraquinone molecular family. This

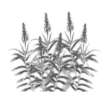

family has specific functions and is used for draining, laxative and purifying purposes. Today, among natural plants, Aloe vera is the most recognized type of plant in this family. This is because the gel found within the leaves of this plant can be easily transformed into pulp and used as a drink or as an ointment for topical purposes. In fact, various molecules possessing herbal therapeutic traits are found in this type of plant, but in less quantity than those present in the smaller leaves of Aloe arborescens.

Aloe and its increased medicinal value: Aloe Arborescens Miller

Compared to Aloe vera, Aloe arborescens has narrower leaves and wider external cuticles that contribute to keeping the plant alive in extreme environmental conditions. This morphologic characteristic allows for a greater presence of anthraquinone elements within the plant, giving it laxative, antiviral and antimicrobic effects. The gel content within Aloe arborescens is proportionally less than Aloe vera. This in turn is less attractive for commercial reasons, forcing Aloe arborescens into a less important position, even though the latter has superior therapeutic qualities than Aloe vera. This was shown in a recent international bibliography.

Aloe arborescens is now being cultivated in Italy, allowing the commercialization of products containing it as a principle ingredient. It is becoming possible to purchase products that have Aloe arborescens as a base ingredient, maintaining the plant's biochemical and hydrotherapeutic characteristics. This is the case in both cosmetic and food products. Due to industrial contamination, the production and use of Aloe vera in Italy has been mostly discontinued. Often, it is imported from other countries at a low qualitative and beneficial level.

Recent studies administered by the Palatinin Salzano Venezia Institute in Italy have discovered that Aloe arborescens is 200% richer in medicinal substances than Aloe vera and contains more than 70% of anti-cancerogenous properties (active ingredients) as opposed to Aloe vera, which contains 40% of these properties.

Aloe throughout the Times

It is practically impossible to separate the legends of the past with what actually happened regarding the use of Aloe in ancient societies. Legends, myths, history and antique research are so intertwined that it is impossible to know where one ends and another begins. In any case, today many of these myths and incorrect facts are active propaganda for some of the most current Aloe information agents.

According to history, the first people to transform Aloe into a commercial extract were the Arabs, which provides a starting point as to when and how Aloe was used on a daily basis. Following the Arabs came the ancient Greek culture, leaving this knowledge of Aloe in Rome, Atlantis, Asia, and Africa. It even made its way to Alessandro Magno (who occupied the island of Socrates and made a point of always having a large supply of Aloe to cure his wounded soldiers during battle). The knowledge of this plant's versatile healing capability moved on to Europe, and then to the Americas via Christopher Columbus.

Today, some still insist on believing that Aloe was brought directly from the Garden of Eden, while other more appropriately informed people maintain that the plant comes from the ancient continent of Atlantis. It is said that the Atlantics possessed various industries in Egypt, Yucatan and the Canaries. This would explain why this plant was present in the past as well as in the Mayan and Toltec civilizations.

For the Mexican native Indians, Aloe remains their sacred protector of excellence. Today, little Mexican shops always have at least one Aloe plant on display. Coincidences exist between ancient Egypt and Mexican pre-Columbian culture, such that international scholars leave one to think that the link between these two cultures could be the disappearance of the Atlantes Island, which was meticulously described by Plato in his works.

The History and Benefits of Aloe

Aloe belongs to the botanical Liliacee family, meaning not the type of plant but the genus of plant that today has been named Aloacee for its more than 350 varieties. We know today that only three or four of these varieties have medicinal properties, including Aloe vera barbadensis and Aloe arborescens. The word Aloe is derived from the Arab word Alloeh, which means "sour substance." It was associated with the Latin word "vera" because in ancient times it was common to consider this type of plant to be more effective in popular medicine. Aloe grows well in tropical climates, such as the hotter regions of America, Asia, Europe and Australia. It prefers a sandy texture to grow in. The Aloe plant is similar to the cactus, for it is capable of retaining large amounts of water to ensure its survival in dry climates.

The Fascinating Story of Aloe as a Natural Remedy for the Egyptians: "The immortal plant"

It is not known the exact period in history when the Aloe plant started to be recognized as a medicinal plant. One of the first documentations of this plant being used as a medicine dates back to 2100 B.C. as found on a piece of clay. However, drawings of this plant have been found in an antique Egyptian temple that dates back to 4000 B.C. Aloe has been forever encircled by a halo of myths and legends, so much so that in some cultures it is considered to be divine, venerated for its healing properties. Whatever the truth may be, it has been historically proven that, dating back to Christ, Aloe has always played a significant pharmaceutical role in antique cultures.

Indisputable proof of the use of this plant exists in regions such as southern Europe, the Orient, Asia and the Americas, etc. One of the most detailed accounts of the earliest uses of Aloe can be found in the Egyptian writing of "Papiro Ebers," dating back to 1550 B.C. This writing documented a series of recipes using Aloe, together with other ingredients, to treat various internal and external ailments. Ancient Egyptians called Aloe "the immortal plant." This explains its use in the embalming process, its importance in the burial rites of pharaohs, and its use by Queen Nefertiti and Queen Cleopatra. Both these beau-tiful women owe their beauty to their daily Aloe baths. It is said that one of Cleopatra's servants would regularly use one of the Queen's creams containing Aloe to be as beautiful as her mistress.

After many years of slavery in Egypt, the Jews adopted various Egyptian funeral rituals and, according to legend, King Solomon appreciated and cultivated his own Aloe for its therapeutic and aromatic agents.

Aloe and the Greeks

The botanical and pharmacological use of Aloe was widely accepted by the Greeks from the Egyptians and Mesopotamians.

Using his aphorisms, recipes, diets, and measuring techniques, the ancient Greek doctor Tippecanoe influenced the Roman world as well as the medieval one. He was the first to organically and systematically classify 300 medicinal plant species.

The philosopher Aristotelico Teofrasto (372-287 B.C.) wrote *Historia Plantarum*, in which he lists all the different varieties of plants in that period, including the Aloe plant.

Pedanio Dioscoride, Greek doctor and naturopath, who originated from Cilicia (modern day Turkey), wrote "De Materia

Medica" (medical matters) while he followed the Roman army in Asia Minor. His work is one of the first authoritative texts that dealt with botany and pharmacology, in which the use of Aloe was fully outlined. Aloe was used to treat ulcers and wounds, insomnia, alopecia, intestinal upsets, constipation, hemorrhoids, gingivitis, bladder problems, burns, etc. Dioscoride had visited the Orient as a military doctor and found Aloe-based remedies useful for 800 clinical conditions. His pharmacology was highly considered among the Arab countries. The respect that Muslims have for Aloe is due to his works. At the same time, in the Latin world, Plinio Il Vecchio (23-79 A.D.) became famous for his work "Naturalis Historia." He confirmed and amplified Dioscoride's theories combining scientific notions with superstitious and magical beliefs.

It is common in today's society to assume that a prescription including Aloe is something of a magic ritual. However, if they carefully examine the prescription, they realize it is a reasonable answer to whatever ailment exists.

For example, when Plinio Il Vecchio recommended that to fight alopecia, one should massage the hair follicles with Aloe juice and alcohol and be in direct sunlight, this was not out of this world. In reality, alcohol together with the sun's heat helps in the opening of the skin's pores, allowing the mixture to penetrate, thus revitalizing the bulb of the hair and stimulating its regrowth.

Galeno (129-210 A.D.) wrote about hypocratic medicinal forms in his Ars Medica. He knew of approximately 500 vegetable-based substances and an array of animal and mineral ones as well. Galeno advocated the "Pica" substance as being one of the best. This substance has Aloe as its principle ingredient.

Another noteworthy reference to Aloe can be found in the New Testament, specifically in the Gospel according to John (Cap. 19, V. 39). He writes that Christ's body had been sprinkled with an oily and aromatic mixture. Recent laboratory studies have discovered traces of Aloe, Mira and plant pollen found in Palestine during those years, thus proving the truthfulness of what was written in the Gospel.

"The silent healer"

In the past, cavalrymen were known to have drunk a mixture of palm wine, Aloe and hemp pulp. This drink was called "elixir" of Jerusalem because it was known to have miraculous capabilities that guaranteed health and longevity. In 600 B.C., Aloe had been introduced into Arab, Persian and Indian markets. The Arabs were clever in discovering the way in which the Aloe plant was to be cultivated to gain medicinal benefits from it. They used it for both external and internal purposes, and the Bedouin tribes and the Tuareg warriors referred to the plant as the "lily of the desert." They separated the plant's gel and lymph from the leaves, folding the leaves with their bare feet. They then poured the pulp onto goatskin, which was set out to dry in the sun. After the process was complete, the pulp was grinded and reduced to powder.

The Indus of the Indus Valley civilization (c3300-1700 B.C.) believed that Aloe grew in the Garden of Eden and named it the silent healer. Ancient Chinese doctors considered the Aloe plant to be endowed with therapeutic properties, and they called it "harmonious remedy."

Appreciated by important ancient people

In America, the Mayan people used the plant for ages. Women used it to hydrate their skin and to wean babies. In Florida, the Seminole Indians believed Aloe was capable in rejuvenating and considered it the "fountain of youth."

The first certain reference to the use of Aloe in the past is in 41-68 B.C. by Dioscoride. He was otherwise known as the Greek herbalist. This doctor gained insight into the use of Aloe while he accompanied the victorious Roman military. He wrote what was considered to be the first detailed description of the Aloe plant. He outlines that the content found in its leaves could have been used for chronic boils, hemorrhoids, to heal foreskin, to prevent dehydration, ulcerated genitals, gingivitis, throat and tonsil inflammation, and to stop hemorrhages.

Plinio Il Vecchio (23-79 A.D.) confirmed Dioscoride's beliefs, but went further to declare that Aloe was useful for many other upsets and was also able in helping to reduce perspiration. The use of Aloe for medicinal purposes gained international acclamation popular during medieval times and the Renaissance. It became increasingly popular in northern Europe, but because this plant grows in mild climates only, it was quickly abandoned.

The constant use of Aloe is also noted by Marco Polo, as well as Christopher Columbus during their travels to Cuba and many Caribbean islands where it was mainly used to cure boils, as well as insect and snake bites. Written in one of Columbus's diaries was the following: "There are four important types of vegetation essential for man's well being. These are grain, grapes, olives and Aloe. The first nurtures, the second brightens one's spirits, the third promotes harmony and the fourth cures."

Almost Supernatural Properties

Knowledge of this "miraculous plant" has been orally passed down from one generation to the next. The various uses of this plant have been written about and archived for years by royal doctors. Priests used it in many religious rites. It isn't a coincidence that Aloe was cited in the Gospel as having been spread across Christ's body after his death. The Jesuits discovered Aloe in the fifteenth century after reading Greek and Latin scientific writings that described its benefits. The Jesuits used the plant they found by chance, cultivating it where no Aloe was to be found. They passed along information regarding the Aloe plant in various American regions. After conquering the natives, the Jesuits founded their mission, promoting the widespread use of Aloe throughout present day Latin America.

"I asked myself what were my secret strengths during my hunger? Yes, it was my undying faith in God, my frugal and simple way of life, and Aloe, realizing its benefits at the end of the XIX century during my arrival in South Africa."

Mahatma Gandhi 1869-1948

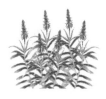

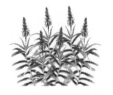

The Chemical Composition of Aloe Arborescens

The use of Aloe for cosmetic, medicinal, nutritional and therapeutic purposes was the result of the enthusiasm regarding this plant and its uses during past centuries, even though its exact chemical composition was not known. As a result of intense and systematic analysis of this plant over the past 40 years, it is now possible to establish the chemical-physical and biochemical-nutritional characteristics of this plant. Work in this field has grown immensely and it is now possible to establish each single biological property of every molecular group that is part of this type of useable plant. Recent studies have promised to enrich the chemical knowledge regarding Aloe. Its results show that Aloe arborescens is made up of a vast series of compounds that can be classified into three large groups:

- **Carbohydrates**, which include polysaccharide mannan (acemannan) and glutens – with immunomodulation;
- **Anthraquinone and phenolic substances** present in the cuticle and leaf, having a laxative, depurative, anti-inflammatory, analgesic and anti-microbiotic effect;
- **Important nutritional and functional molecules**, such as mineral salts, vitamins, amino acids, organic acids, lipids (polyunsaturated fatty acids) and enzymes.

The average percentage composition in the natural chemical components of the Aloe arborescens per 100 g. of s.s. This is

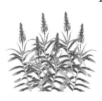

about 7% protein, 2% lipids, 22% ashes (includes all the diverse mineral elements of the plant), 70% carbohydrates (which contribute to numerous types of complex and simple glycids) and finally, a quantitative but not relevant percentage (but biologically important) of vitamins present (free amino acids and all other organically natural molecules with chemically different characteristics). These represent a part of the diverse active ingredients, biologically effective and characteristically part of the Aloe species.

Water is characterized as the largest component in Aloe. It makes up approximately 96% of its fresh weight and is distributed throughout 90% of the plant's cuticle and 98% of the trimming of the plant's leaves, whereas it makes up 99% of the plant's essence.

Carbohydrates Found in Aloe Arborescens

Carbohydrates are organic molecules that are most diffused throughout plants. Primarily, they are found in vegetation, where all plants present a qualitative pool of similarities. Nevertheless, some of them can be differentiated by the presence of specific molecules of this class.

Monosaccharide

Simple glycids are found in the Aloe plant, particularly glucose and magnesium. They make up roughly 10% to 25% of the dry variable within the diverse components of the leaves, cuticles, veins, and essence. The glucose represents more than

95% of the total soluble glycid amount. The remaining fractions are composed of other types of non-important glycids. Glucose is metabolically glycidic, our bodies use it, and it's important our energy level is based on this nutrient.

Polysaccharide

Numerous types of polysaccharides are present in Aloe with exceptionally high concentrations. The most important polysaccharide with respect to hydrotherapeutic activity is acemannan. This substance is the majority substance found throughout the cells of the leaves.

The percentage of polysaccharide in Aloe is important for the cosmetic and hydro pharmaceutical industries. For topical use, this macro-molecule guarantees an appropriate application of water on the skin, forming a semi-permeable base that causes hydration of the skin, leaving it soft and elastic. When swallowed, mannan properties are absorbed not at a gastro-enteric level, but rather at an intestinal mucus level, allowing endocitosis. They are capable of strengthening an organism's immune system, activating the lymphocytes and macrophage cells needed for fagocitic activities, capable of eliminating strange and toxic material in the organism. The acemannan performs bacterial and anti-fungal activities. It also is known for its ability to form gel and protecting gastric and intestinal mucus from damaging agents like chloric acid and gastric acid.

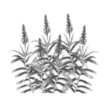

Anthraquinone Molecules

Molecules consisting of anthraquinone chemicals make up a vast group of substances that possess numerous hydro-therapeutic properties. The regulatory actions on intestinal motility are clearly recognized with the increase of peristalsis and with laxative effects. The principal molecules of this group are: Aloemodin, Aloin, Aleolithic, Antranol, Crysophanic acid and Resistanolo. Most of these products are recognized within the pharmaceutical family and are used to create laxatives and digestives. In people who are extremely sensitive to medicine, it is common to experience diarrhea when beginning to take Aloe. This condition usually disappears in a few days. It is for this reason many producers of food containing Aloe vera deprive the Aloe gel within the anthraquinone level of its ability to filter the active carbon.

It should be noted that this procedure also removes another important component useful for hydrotherapeutic purposes and also anthraquinone properties that modulate the different physiologic choices the body can use for self-deprivation. To eliminate the inconvenience caused by the use of carbon filtering, it would be advisable to keep the anthraquinone properties, monitoring their exact presence level. This way, their important anti-bacterial and antiviral properties can be used, causing citotoxic effects on tumorous cells characterized in some anthra-quinone molecules.

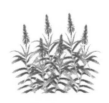

Aleolithic Acid

This molecule represents a natural antibiotic action, particularly in association with other anthraquinone molecules present in Aloe.

Cinnamic Acid

Chemical product having intense antibiotic, antibacterial and germicidal effects needed to combat various bacteria, including salmonella, streptococci and staphylococci. The bacteria that cause peptic ulcers have been proven to be inhibited by this product. The hydrotherapeutic properties of this molecule, being of a phenolic nature, include the inflammation process and the defense against UV rays.

Crysophanic Acid

This molecule is also of anthraquinone nature and presents similar properties to those described for this group of molecule. It is a good purifying, diuretic and laxative agent, having eupeptic and tonifying properties.

Aloemodin

This is an anthraquinone molecule that originates from aloin, resulting from a division from a glycoside relationship producing an arsines and Aloemodin liberation. This molecule has important citotoxic effects on specific predaceous and cancerous cells

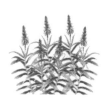

Aloin

This is a principle agent exclusively present in Aloe and is made up of different anthraquinone glycoside derivatives. It is present in the form of two isometric indicators, such as Aloin A and B, and is the wildcard molecular denomination that better represents this class of composts. Other denominations are used when its exact origin from other forms of Aloe is indicated. For this, the molecule is indicated in parabolic terms if it is derived from Aloe barbadensis, Socaloin if it is derived from Socotrin Aloe, etc. This molecule has antibiotic, puritive and laxative agents.

Phenolic Compositions

The fraction of molecules being of phenolic nature and having antioxidant effects consist of Cinnamic acid derivatives, cumarinic molecules, flavinoids, polyfunctional organic acids and tocopherols. These molecules play an important role in contrasting free radicals and oxygen-reactive species that are responsible for numerous negative effects on the body. A classic example of this is the aging process. Various phonological composts within the Aloe plant have been highlighted within the cumarinic group of molecules and present in the form of glycosides. These molecules show intense antioxidant activity, similar to that of tocopherols. Aloeresine A and B are phenolic-natured molecules present in Aloe arborescens.

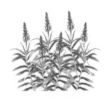

Salicylic Acid

This substance is vital in the making of aspirin. With regards to Aloe's essence, this acid performs antiseptic, painkiller and anti-inflammatory functions.

Other Components

Other molecules and hydrotherapeutic activities are present in Aloe arborescens, among them sterol, vegetables, triterpen, saponines and lignin.

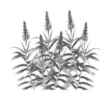

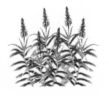

Nutrients Present in Aloe

The Aloe plant appears to be qualitatively rich in vitamins and in mineral salts, even if their quantity is modest. This allows Aloe's essence to be pure, making it comparable to nutritional supplements containing a high concentration of vitamins and minerals. It is proportionally balanced and optimal for regulatory effects produced by this product.

Mineral Salts

The Aloe plant has numerous macro-elemental minerals. These include calcium, magnesium, potassium and sodium. These elements are most commonly found, yet there are other less common elemental minerals that also are present in Aloe. These oligoelements serve a particular function in the organism and include magnesium, iron, copper, zinc, and chrome. It is important that all macro elements are present within an organism and function in conjunction with one another to maintain an appropriate functioning relationship between them.

Sodium

Sodium is a fundamental mineral found within the organism's liquid content. It is found in cation form and is associated with ion, chloride or bicarbonate. Sodium is the most characteristic cation within extracellular liquids and is capable of regulating the osmotic processes within this section of the organism's

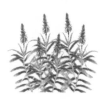

liquid content. It is important in maintaining the aqueous saline balance and has to be present in properly defined quantities. Together with calcium, this element has an important role on the micardic properties. In the form of sodium choride, sodium stimulates appetite and helps in the digestion process with the secretion of gastric juices and with chloric acid.

Potassium

This element is most widely present within the intracellular liquid in cation form and is associated with chloric ion. It participates in intracellular osmotic processes and is an important element needed for muscle tissue. It possesses excitatory phenomenon that include the body's nerves, heart, both streaked and relaxed muscles, and endocrine glands. An insufficient supply of potassium could result in many malformations, including cavities, bronchitis, circulatory pain, acne, colds and a much slower healing process for wounds. In the case of hypoglycemia, the delicate relationship between potassium and sodium is in jeopardy thus giving rise to a serious imbalance of the hydria saline.

Calcium

Calcium is the most represented mace element in our body. It makes up 2% of our total body weight mainly as a component in our bone density. Like catione, it is present in both extra-cellular and intracellular sections of our body. It has an important biochemical and physiological function. Having numerous enzymes dependent on calcium and on biochemical and physiological processes, this mineral is the modulator for the metabolic paths, including the coagulation of the blood, muscular contractions, the functioning of the nervous system and of the heart. Aloe contains approximately 5% of the dry weight total of a leaf.

Magnesium

Directly related to calcium, this mineral element is present in bivalent cation form and is abandoned in the intracellular liquids where it acts upon many enzymatic systems. Like calcium, it is present within the bones and occupies approximately 50% of the total magnesium found within the organism. It is vital for muscular growth, individual vitality and especially enzyme functioning involved with cellular oxidization. It is an important factor in the immunological system and its weakening provokes bacterial and viral aggression on the body. It is involved with synaptic nerve transmission and has calming and anti-depressive functions. It ranks fourth with respect to mineral content, making up 0.8% of the dry weight within the Aloe.

Oligoelements

The oligoelements just slightly present make up less of a percentage within the living organism, yet they perform regulatory functions needed for metabolic regularity. There fails to be a direct correlation between the slightly present elements and microelements that make up a larger percentage of the total. Usually, the practice is to classify the oligoelements present in the body's tissue on a basis of one thousand or in concentration inferior to this number. Generally, all the elements found within a living organism's environment can be assumed, so that all of the elements just barely present within an organism ought to be numbered or almost all those elements that are known. In reality, it is vital that these minimally present elements are existent because they perform the necessary functions for survival or at least for the organism's well being. In most cases, these elements perform catalytic functions via the combination of molecular proteins. These barely present elements are essential components to various enzymatic systems. Many of them react on the basis of their capabilities in forming complex formations of enzymatic proteins they contain.

Manganese

It is chemically similar to magnesium but has different functions with respect to the organism. It has high antioxidant powers and contributes to the slowing down of the aging process. It is principally found in the liver and in muscle tissue. It is important for breastfeeding children and for natal development. A deficiency of this mineral may cause excessive irritability, convulsions and vessel dilation. It is directly related to calcium and potassium with respect to metabolism.

Iron

Iron is inappropriately considered an oligoelement because our bodies contain 5g of it and it is too much to consider this

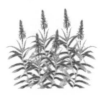

element as having just a trace quantity. Its importance within the body is very well known. It is needed for both the external and cellular respiratory process, belonging to the prosthetic hemoglobin and cytocromic groups. Iron present in one's diet is intestinally absorbed. Almost the entire digestive system is capable of this absorption. For this reason, the ferrous form is preferred as opposed to the ferric and ascorbic acid because it may bring an increase in the absorption of this mineral. Various dietetic factors may result in a decrease of this mineral's absorption, causing anemia.

Copper

Copper is an important element for the well being of organisms. The liver contains a major concentration of this mineral (6,6 g/g of tissue), followed by the brain (5,4 g/g of tissue). The average quantity of copper found within vertebra organisms is about 1,5-2,5 g/g of lean tissue. In total, approximately 100-130 mg of copper are present within the human body. Copper is necessary for adequate erythropoiesis (the process to form red blood cells), perhaps because it is required for the release of iron into the tissues. It is also necessary for connective tissue maturation.

This mineral enters into various enzymatic constitutions that are generally involved with the catalase oxyoreduction. The lack of copper within one's body prohibits the absorption of calcium and phosphate into bone mass. In addition, a lack of this mineral determined by normal catalase conditions prohibits the accumulation of oxygenized water, thus resulting in self-intoxication. According to some scholars, cancerous states could result from a decrease of catalase activity.

Zinc

Two to three grams of our body are made up of zinc, and it is primarily found in the liver and pancreas. It is fundamental for the proper functioning of various enzymes. This mineral has an important nutritional role. The degree of carbohydrate and protein absorption into the body depends on the level of zinc found in the body.

Chrome

Generally, animals have a very low level of this mineral in their systems, approximately 0.1 ppm. Chrome is scarcely absorbed in the intestines, allowing for only 0.5-3% of regular chrome intake unabsorbed into an organism. It is eliminated via urination and feces. With respect to the plasma, chrome is transported from the transferrins in the same way as iron. The biochemical function of this mineral seems to be related to insulin and to the transportation of cellular metabolites through to the cellular membranes. Insulin requires the presence of chrome to perform its duties. Without insulin, chrome cannot have an insulin-based effect on the organism.

Cobalt

This oligoelement is minimally present in the human body

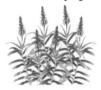

(approx. 20 mg) and is concentrated in the spleen, pancreas and liver. The lack of this mineral may cause a reduction in the content of hemoglobin in the blood. It is part of the B12 structure and reacts to erythropoiesis (the natural process of production of red blood cells that occurs in the bone marrow) and allows for protein and carbohydrate regulation of the metabolism.

Vitamins

These molecules are needed for the biological functioning of living organisms. They are nutritionally essential and must be introduced into the body via food intake or in pro vitamin form that is non-synthesizable by our cellular systems. Perhaps the total amount of vitamins obtained directly or indirectly by animals is capable of being synthesized. These molecules perform a regulatory function with respect to cellular metabolism. The water-soluble vitamins make up various indispensable co-enzymatic forms needed for numerous enzymatic activities, while those classified fat-soluble perform other types of actions, though always along regulatory lines, including hormonal activities (Vitamin D is a precursor to a hormone action molecule). The availability of vitamin-based nutrients ensures an optimal level of health, while a lack of vitamins caused by food intake or an alteration in the organism's functions can cause particular and specific pathological states. In extreme cases, it may even cause death. An excess intake of water-soluble vitamins will not cause any detrimental effects, but an excessive intake of fat-soluble vitamins, meaning Vitamins A and D, can be toxic. When it comes to nutrition, it is advisable to assure an accurate vitamin intake by consuming foods that will replenish and balance various vitamin factors as opposed to resorting to medicinal ones.

The Aloe arborescens plant presents discrete vitamin content. It can be qualitatively and quantitatively appreciated.

The following list outlines the vitamins present in this plant and a brief explanation of the biological activities of each of these vitamins.

Water-Soluble Vitamins

Vitamin B1 or Thiamine

Constitutes an important co-enzymatic form of enzymes involved in energetic cellular metabolism. It is fundamental for the growth process of body tissue and for the proper functioning of the nervous system. A lack of this vitamin may cause severe anemia, neuritis and edema.

Vitamin B2 or Riboflavin

Participates in cellular respiration and in the replenishment of the organism energy level. A lack of this vitamin may cause dermatitis and hematological ulcerations.

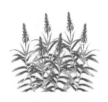

Vitamin B3 or Niacin

Regulates metabolic energy and participates in the process of glucose use. A lack of this vitamin may cause pellagra.

Vitamin B6 or Pyridoxine

Constitutes all the co-enzymes of all enzymatic activity proposed by the use of amino acids. It regulates the nervous system, contributing to the functioning of the skin.

Vitamin C or Ascorbic Acid

Perhaps the best-known vitamin. In high dosages, it continues to perform preemptory actions with respect to the common cold to microorganism infections. It is also internationally used to fight against common cold symptoms. It helps to fight against antioxidant and free anti-radicals. It is an effective protective agent for the organism, promoting tissue growth, wound healing, and polysaccharides synthesis and collagen formation. It maintains the mucous function and is essential for bone and tooth formation. Lack of this vitamin promotes scurvy.

Folic Acid

This vitamin is present in all green leaves and is found in human liver and kidneys. Under co-enzymatic form, it participates in numerous reactions that involve mutilation of various vital molecules for the organism, such as thiamine, a DNA component. Together with B12, it is useful as an anti-anemic vitamin. Lack of this vitamin may cause megoblastic anemia.

Cholene (Vitamin B Group)

An organic compound that is a necessary nutrient. In reality, it can't be considered a true vitamin because it can be synthesized within the organism. In any case, it performs specific roles. It's the precursor to acetylcholine, a neuron-transmitter, and performs functions relating to mobilization mechanisms and aids in the transportation of bodily lipids. Lack of this vitamin may cause fat infiltration into the liver.

Fat-Soluble Vitamins

Vitamin A and Retinol

This vitamin is not present in vegetation, but it is quantitatively represented in various forms. Carotene is an example of this. This vitamin factor intervenes throughout numerous cellular metabolic processes. It is involved in the mucopolysaccharide synthesis mechanisms and in the proteic synthesis process, as well. It contributes to cellular membrane stability, namely mitochondrion and lisosomes. It performs a specific biochemical function regarding sight. Lack of Vitamin A determines night blindness, dryness and desquamation (peeling) of the skin and increases the chance of infections.

Vitamin E or Tocopherols

This vitamin is a potent antioxidant. It protects membranic lipids from oxidant processes, free radicals and from reactive oxygen reactions. It is associated with the skin's well being, tissue growth (namely the liver, kidneys, intestines and genitals). It promotes the production of bone marrow. Lack of this vitamin may cause skin ulcers, anemia and bone malformations. High doses of this vitamin help fight infection. Various experimental results show the effectiveness of this vitamin against carcinogenic agents. It has always been considered effective in respiratory insufficiency, in pneumonia and in asthma cases. A good quantity of this vitamin is found in the gel of the Aloe arborescens leaf.

Protein

The content of protein in Aloe is comparable in terms to other vegetation. It represents 7% of dry weight, considering that 96-97% of the Aloe leaf is made up of water. This quantity of Aloe is not regarded as being elevated. The protein component in the Aloe is nevertheless important for two reasons; a) the presence of determining enzymes within the cellular structure of the leaf that perform specific functions and which are involved in hydrotherapeutic aspects of some digestive actions, and b) the various proteins present in the Aloe after their digestion contribute to the refurbishing of amino acids, even if it is quantitatively limited for our bodies.

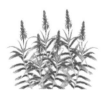

Enzymes

Enzymes are protein-natured molecules that allow for the development of all vital functions within a cell, increasing reactional velocity that characterizes cellular metabolism. In their presence, all biochemical reactions happen immediately. Most importantly, these reactions are compatible with life. The most important enzymes are the following:

- **Bradykininase** – it is a proteolysis nature's enzyme that in a specific way catalyzes bradykinin peptic molecular degradation. This peptic is capable of stimulating an inflammatory response to an allergenic agent that enters our bodies. For example, this can happen through an open wound. Bradykinin is responsible for pain and post-traumatic tumescence of the tissue. Bradykininase enzymes contained in Aloe stimulate the immune system by activating local macrophages. It performs an analgesic, anti-inflammatory and wound healing function, degrading the bradykinin.

- **Catalase** – this enzyme deals with the degradation of oxygenized water that is formed in some metabolic reactions in which it has a toxic effect, activating free radicals. When using Aloe for topical reasons, the catalase could act as a detergent in burn and ulceration cases, favoring scarring and thus introducing fibro-blast production. Amylase, cellulose, lipase, carboxypeptidases and other protease are other enzymes present in Aloe that can be placed in this classification. These enzymes can help with the digestive system, contributing to the degradation of vitamins assimilated via food intake.

- **Amino acids** – these molecules make up the unit base of protein. There are 20 types of these molecules. Nutritionally speaking, some of these are more important than others because they are not produced within the body itself. To replenish the body with these, we must ensure that we are properly nourishing ourselves. Aloe helps the body replenish itself with amino acids, especially the essential ones, even though the amount of absolute protein is relatively low.

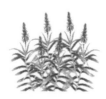

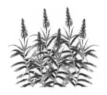

Aloe Arborescens:
A Healthy Contribution from a Usable Plant

Biological and Herbal Therapeutic
Characteristics

Aloe has many biological and herbal therapeutic properties, as proven by the extensive research done this past century. This research has characterized the use of this plant in greater depth than what was thought many years ago. Aloe's properties allow it to be used for a vast array of small and large pathologies in which its active components are used. Today, scientific literature discusses many different pathologies that may occur in our bodies for which the use of Aloe is appropriate. Aloe has been used for herbal therapeutic as well as for health concerns, as documented in medical-scientific journals. Animal and controlled laboratory research has proven the effectiveness of Aloe for various pathologies and these results have been published in international biomedical journals. In addition, you will find Aloe in common households being used as a topical cure for small ailments. American and South American researchers support a school of thought that believes in the herbal therapeutic properties of Aloe, referring exclusively to the acemannan polysaccharide molecules. American Aloe-based products commonly eliminate Aloin as well as other principal agents. We should note that the positive effects of Aloe on the body depend on a coordinated use of the product, not only the present poly-saccharides but also the other molecules. The herbal therapeutic properties of some of these molecules are widely recognized in the official pharmacopoeia and in biochemical research. There is a very important synergistic role between amino acids, vitamins, mineral salts, glycids, polyunsaturated fats and certain enzymes.

With its botanical attributes, biochemical composition and biological characteristics, it is important to consider that Aloe possesses a variety of herbal therapeutic properties.

Recognized Antioxidant Properties

Antioxidant properties biochemically belong to all those chemically diverse molecules, in that they are capable of neutralizing numerous nitrogen and oxygenic free radicals, as well as the species that react to oxygen that are responsible for molecular and subcellular alterations, thus causing the onset of the aging and precancerous processes. Anti-oxidant molecules present in Aloe arborescens are numerous and include magnesium and copper, Vitamins B2, C and E, and anthraquinone and phenolic molecules. Magnesium and copper are active constituents of the superoxydic and peroxidasic glutatonic enzymes that perform antioxidant and anti-aging actions for the body as well as the skin. Similarly, Vitamin B2 permits the maintenance of a high cellular level of reduced glutton, the anti-radical molecule. Vitamin C is a typical antioxidant in the intracellular environment (especially regarding white blood cells), while the same function is administered by Vitamin E with respect to cellular membranes lipids. Even anthraquinone and phenolic molecules are effective antioxidant agents. Therefore, the use of Aloe guarantees an appropriate agent molecular consistency that enhances the body's antioxidant reserves and fights cellular and tissue aging.

Peculiar Anti-Aging Properties

More than just an antioxidant property, Aloe arborescens helps maintain the youthfulness of the skin. This is thought to be as result of the plant's capacity to increase the production and growth of fibroblast up to 6-8 times. These derma-localized cells are responsible for the production of collagen. Collagen is a protein that leaves the skin soft and elastic. During the aging process, these cells reduce collagen production, leaving the skin with less elasticity and more dryness, resulting in wrinkles.

Aloe is capable of increasing fibroblast production, increasing the production of collagen. The key to this process is tied to Aloe's polysaccharide action on fibroblast multiplication and to their hydrating properties. These effects tend to rejuvenate the skin, reorganizing its normal tegumental look and reducing the visible lines of aging.

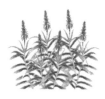

Evident Antibacterial, Antimicrobic and Antiviral Properties

Specific molecules included in Aloe arborescens sustain each of these properties. Aloe is capable of retarding the development of bacteria and fungi because of the presence of two organic acids: Cinnamic and Crysophanic. Their citotoxic characteristics are due to their anthraquinone components within the molecule, which affects the patogeneous cellular agents. In particular, Crysophanic acids have a positive action on fungi, which can easily enter our bodies via the intestines. In addition to being a fungicide, this molecule has a laxative and depurative effect as well. Simply, it allows for the removal of toxic waste produced within our intestines. The antibiotic property is given to Aloe via the presence of glycosides.

Glycosides are considered to be an anthraquinone structure that is similar to aloetic acid and Aloin and contributes acemannan polysaccharide and Bradykininase enzymes. This enzyme is particularly presented within the Aloe arborescens. All these factors put together result in the activation and participation of macrophage and interleukin production on the immune system.

Specific Anti-Inflammatory and Anti-Pain Properties

Throughout past centuries of Aloe usage, anti-inflammatory and anti-pain properties are perhaps its most known and appreciated herbal therapeutic characteristics. Its calming and soothing actions are similar to steroid-based anti-inflammatory medicines without the collateral effects. Aloe's active anti-inflammatory components can be identified in three vegetable steroidal-based molecules: composterol, sitosterol and luteol. These three molecules act to inhibit the prostaglandin's effects. Aloe's effective and immediate control on the swelling process is also a result of the acemannan and its Brabykininase. The first activates the phagocytes and the second determines the brandikin's degradation and other interleukin, which in turn are liberated from the swelling process. This intense activity produced within a body's swelling components has anti-pain and soothing effects. These effects contribute to the salicylic acid and anthraquinone molecules. Similarly, this effect is also experienced with Cinnamic acid and isobarboloin, which are also components of Aloe arborescens' active ingredients.

Cicatrizing (Wound Healing) Characteristic Properties and Epithelial Stimulated Growth

With respect to wound healing, Aloe's cicatrizing properties date back to Alessandro Magno. Whether used topically or administered orally, Aloe's positive healing effects are partly related to the plant's anti-inflammatory capabilities. The principal characteristics of the plant produce diverse mechanisms that are involved in the positive processes. This is caused by an inhibition reaction in the anti-inflammatory process and in the stimulatory reaction in the cicatrizing process. The stimulatory effects occur on typical cells, which are important to skin formation, such as fibroblast, cheratinocit and derma cells. Particular importance is seen in the functioning of the fibroblast used in collagen production, which plays a fundamental role in the formation of fibrosis wounds together with other extracellular matrix components. There are two ways in which Aloe participates in the cicatrizing process. One is via the elevated molecular acemannan. The second is via the low-weighted and vegetable-based steroid anthraquinone. In this content, the acemannan stimulates the macrophage's activity by chemically signaled production that affects cellular proliferation. This is particularly true for the fibroblasts, which are also involved in the final wound-healing phase, favoring riepitelization. The acemannan molecules then inhibit development of various wound microorganisms, which include actions that are equally administered in other molecules. Various low-weighted molecular composts are in many ways involved within the cicatrizing mechanism. Some of these composts are capable of stimulating the angiogenesis processes. These processes are necessary for tissue regeneration and revascularization. Other low-weighted molecular components, like Cinnamic and Crysophanic acid perform very important control functions on infectious wound processes. It is important to mention that the observation of the positive effects found on wounds is closely related to the use of fresh Aloe products. This is because certain treatments may alter various active molecules, resulting in the loss of potential herbal therapeutic benefits.

Surprising Immunomodulatory Properties

The interactional mechanism between elevated weighted molecular components holds an important role in numerous vital processes, intending to maintain the body's internal environmental integrity. Polysaccharides or glycoprotein-natured molecules are involved in such activities, particularly regarding the immune system. The defense mechanism's effectiveness against external elements is certainly tied to the proper functioning of the immune system. This is for both its absolute potentiality and when it is capable of responding according to the circumstance.

In various pre-pathologic or conclamate characterized pathologic situations, an individual's immune system may fluctuate from an initial functional alteration to a strong immunological reduction potential. This may cause serious pathological consequences. The acemannan performs the immunomodulatory properties in Aloe arborescens (similar to the glucans). The acemannan has a protective effect on organisms. Aloe contains the highest concentration of this vegetable-based molecule. Arborescens slightly varies in that it is a biologically more active form. Acemannan actively stimulates the lymphocytes response. The response reaction appears to be specific for the acemannan, as opposed to other polysaccharides and the effect is aimed at t-cell production and macrophage activity, creating strong interleukin production with strong immunogenic activities. These actions, which result in the modulation and strengthening of the immune system, are related to polysaccharidic-natured molecules without peptic components. It is important to note that natural glycol-protein products such as lectin aloetina A & B from Aloe arborescens have been found in Aloe itself. These products seem to be involved in the strengthening of the immune system, thus inhibiting "in vivo" attributes from the fibro sarcoma and other tumoral-cell growth.

Singular Hypoglycemic Properties

Numerous experimental and epidemiological observations of fresh Aloe leaves have shown a positive hypoglycemic effect in both patients with diabetes mellitus and insulin-dependent diabetics. This effect is attained by polysaccharide fractions of watery Aloe arborescens extracts. In particular, two acemannan fractions called Erboran A & B have proven to be effective in achieving a severe glycemic reduction in both diabetic patients and rats. It is important to note that the administration of Aloe arborescens to diabetic patients allows for the healing of diabetic-associated ulcerations.

Possible Anti-Tumor Properties

Numerous articles based on the medical benefits of Aloe have and are continuing to scientifically demonstrate Aloe's therapeutic and anti-tumor potential. A vast but prudent bibliography demonstrating anti-tumor effects of various Aloe components on precancerous and cancerous in vitro cells and on real experimental animal neoplasis is now available. This action seems to be tied to the acemannan immune-stimulant properties and glycoprotein up to anthraquinone antiviral and citotoxic properties. It is also related to anthraquinone and phenolic antioxidant and free radical effects as well as antioxidant vitamins (beta-carotene, Vitamin C and tocopherols) ending with the role of oligoelements. Some examples of scientific literature on Aloe's phytotherapeutic (plant therapy) potentials are present in the following citation of specific bibliographic references.

(a) In laboratory experimentation on cancerous and pre-cancerous cells.

Research has been done on Aloe's anti-tumor activities. This research has been administered on cultured leukemic human and animal cells and in neuroectodermal cultured cells. The results were very encouraging, in that they demonstrated Aloe's intense cytotoxic inhibition activities in the development of the usual tumor cells.

- Gribel, A. Pahinskii, K. 1986. Antimetastic properties of Aloe juice. Voposy onkologii, 32, (12), 38-40

- Jeong-he-yun, et al. Anticancer effects of Aloe on sarcoma 180 in IRC mouse and on human cancer lines. Yakhak Hoechi. 38, (3), 311-321

- Lee. K.H., Kim, J. H., D. S., Kim C. H., 2000. Anti-leukemia and anti-mutagenic effects of (2.ethylhexyl)phthalate isolated from Aloe vera Linne J. Pharm. Phatmacol, 52, 593598

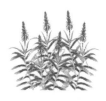

- Pecere, T., et al., 2000. Aloe-emodin is a new type of anticancer agent with selective activity against neuro-ectodermal tumors. Cancer Res. 60, 2800-2804

- Winters, A. et al., 1981. Effects of Aloe on human normal and tumors cells in vitro. Econ. Bot. 35, 89-95

(b) Observations on antitumoral effects on experimental animals

Numerous publications have appeared with respect to Aloe's antitumoral and antimetasis effects on various types of animal-induced tumors. The results showed positive derivatives from Aloe supplementation when it achieves:

1) the reduction in the heptacarcinogeneses (liver tumor) severity on rats;

2) inhibition in tumor reduction with cancerogenous materials in rats;

3) the arrest and regression of fibrosaracoma growth in cats;

4) carcinogen inhibition on rat liver;

5) the reduction of experimental subjects mortality who are infected with Norman sarcoma;

6) phytotherapeutic effect on pleura rat tumors.

The outcome of these results derived from Aloe in 1991 has allowed American approved health officials to use acemannan in curing dog and cat fibrosaracoma where past cures were non-

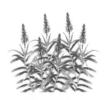

existent.

- Corsi, M.M., et al, 1998. The therapeutic potential of Aloe vera in tumor-bearing rats. Int. J. Tissue React. 20, 115-118 (c) Clinical Studies.

- Harris, C., Pierce, K., King, G., Yates, K.M., Hall, J., Tizzard, I., 1991. Efficacy of acemannan in treatment of canine and feline spontaneous neoplasms. Molecular Biotherapy 3, 207-213.

- Imanishi, K., Ishiguro, T., Saito, H., Suzuki, I., 1981. Pharmacological studies on plant lectin, Aloctin A. I Growth inhibition of mouse methyl-cholanthrene-induced fibrosarcoma (Meth A) in ascites form by Aloctin A. Experientia 37, 1186-1187

- Peng, S.Y., Norman, J., Curtin. G., Corrier, D., McDaniel, H.R., Busbee, D., 1991. Decreased mortalità of Norman murin sarcoma in mice treated with the immunomodulator, acemannan. Molecular Biotherapy 3, 79-87

- Prng, A., et al, USA 1991. Decrease in mouse mortality rates for Norman Sarcoma, treated with immuno-modulatory acemannan. Anatomy Department, Veterinary Medical School, University of Texas.

- Tsuda, H., Ito, M., Girono, I., Kawai, K., Beppu, H., Fujita, K., Nagao, M., 1993. Inhibitory effect of Aloe Arborescens Miller on induction of preneoplastic focal lesions in the rat liver. Phytotherapy Research 7, S43-S47

- Yagi, A., Makino, K., Nishioka, I., Kuchino, Y., 1977. Aloe mannan, polysaccharide from Aloe arborescens var. natalensis. Planta medica 31, 17-20

Epidemiologic studies in the diffusion of human lung tumors in subjects who smoke showed that the consumption of Aloe juice prevents lung carcinogensis and stomach and colon tumors.

- Inahata, K., Nakasugu, T. 1995. Mutagenesis inhibitors. Japanese Patent. JP 7053397.

- Pecere, T., et al. 2000. Aloe-emodin is a new type of anti-cancer agent with selective activity against neuro-ectodermal tumors. Cancer Res. 60, 2800-2804

- Sakai, R., 1989. Epidemiologic survey on lung cancer with respect to cigarette smoking and plant diet. Japanese Journal of Cancer Research 80, 513-520

Other important observations and testimonies on the therapeutic effects of Aloe on important subjects like neoplase, which represent the second cause of death in Italy, were published in specific scientific texts. These observations represent a valid aspect of this plant's use for anti-tumoral remedies, even if they have yet to be clinically or experimentally proven.

Father Romano Zago, OFM, 2003.
Di Cancro si può guarire (Cancer is curable).

Healthy Therapeutic Effects of Aloe Arborescens Found in Scientific Literature

Aloe's list of biological and herbal therapeutic properties is surprisingly extensive. Many misinformed people ask themselves how it is possible that this completely usable plant represents: the most potent natural non-intoxicating agents, the most effective immune system stimulator and regulator, a valid anti-inflammation agent, an analgesic, an antiseptic, a tissue-regenerate stimulator, a skin healer, an anti-intoxicant and anti-age remedy, and a skin protector. All of these factors have been biomedically experimented and proven. The attached bibliography illustrates Aloe's diverse qualities. In addition, it can be said that each of the numerous natural molecules that are included in Aloe arborescens' rich collection have specific herbal therapeutic properties. These plant properties are highlighted for their reciprocal synergic actions of both usable components and nutritional factors. These herbal therapeutic characteristics make Aloe a potent remedy for numerous severe and less severe pathologies that can include diverse organs and other parts of the organism.

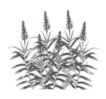

Digestive System

Aloe arborescens' principal properties are capable of having healthy effects on the digestive system. Aloe is used in mouthwash or gel form to act as a mucous protector, lesion corrector, anti-inflammatory agent; it produces an antimicotic and antimicrobic effect, and it normalizes oral pH levels and fights halitosis.

Regarding the stomach, Aloe arborescens' enriched mucopolisaccharides allow for the development of: a) valid stomach mucous protection against gastric acids by inhibiting chloridic acid protection, b) wound healing properties that inhibit helicobacter pylori growth; and c) anti-inflammatory action with lenitive effects on gastritis and on the esophagus. Aloe's Colina, inositol, zinc and selenium contents help with hepatic insufficiencies by intervening in the hepatic cellular membrane fluid and in metabolic processes, thus resolving part of the body's functional difficulties. In particular, Aloe is an effective intestine control remedy for the following symptoms:

1) Lazy bowel and constipation, increasing intestinal peristalsis by using mucillagin and hemicelluloses actions;

2) Colitis and intestine-related pathologies. In this case, it is used as an anti-inflammatory, lenitive and wound healer;

3) Diarrhea: Aloe can resolve this intestinal malfunction because of its nutritional, anti-bacterial, antiseptic and anti-inflammatory components;

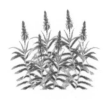

4) Fights dangerous flora bacterial settlement, but it's also effective against microorganisms as: salmonella, streptococci and staphylococci. It is used to fight against candida albicans intestinal mucous. The anthraquinone component is also sustained by the acemannan's immuno-stimulating effect. It is non-toxic to the body and maintains the entire digestive system effectively.

Integument System

Another effective therapeutic action by Aloe. It has been popular since antiquity and is used primarily for skin pathologies. Even in this case, Aloe is considered to be a multi-purpose plant, because its principal active ingredients are capable of resolving numerous skin conditions, such as acne, acne rosacea, pimples, dermatitis and eczema. Aloe arborescens offers a wide array of principal ingredients as well as benefits useful for metabolic functional conditions, infections and inflammations.

The use of Aloe arborescens' pure gel and other cosmetic products is important because it is capable of protecting the skin. Cosmetics with Aloe stimulate the blood flow, guaranteeing an improved level of beneficial activities and the capacity to eliminate Aloe prepared cosmetics toxins. The skin then appears elevated, hydrated and elastic, invigorating its antioxidant defense system to fight free radicals and degenerative actions on the epithelia. This produces an anti-aging and rejuvenating effect. Aloe's excellent capabilities to heal wounds can be used to speed the wound marginization process, sunburns, heat wounds, radiation and bruises.

Cardio-Circulatory System

Aloe arborescens can have a positive effect on this system. In addition to being an effective cleaner or toxin eliminator, the various Aloe components can determine the existence of Hemitrope process, thus resolving anemia. It can have a positive effect on headaches, tiredness and muscular aches. Finally, Aloe's composition includes an elevated quantity of edible fiber, vitamins and polyunsaturated antioxidant components. Aloe is useful as a prevention technique and as a lipidic material depositor for arteries and as an aid to atheromatosis and arteriosclerosis processes. It is also used as a topical remedy and other forms that allow Aloe to effectively fight varicose veins and the loss of elasticity in the skin. In addition, Aloe's immunomodulatory, anti-inflammatory and analgesic actions are due to the acemannans, anthraquinones and vitamins that help fight against lunatics-associated inflammatory reactions.

Immune System

The immuno-stimulating and immunomodulating muco-polysaccharide agents, such as mannan, acemannans and glucans, found in Aloe arborescens make this plant the most important remedy for numerous immune system malfunctions.

Often, the use of Aloe may resolve the following pathologies:

Rheumatoid Arthritis

This pathology is characterized by severe inflammation. It causes severe functional and anatomic complications, antigen and antibody deposits, inflammation and pain. The prolonged use of Aloe arborescens-based products is effective in fighting the effects of this pathology.

Vaginal Candida

The disturbing itchiness caused by Candida albicans is effectively controlled by the topical use of Aloe-based products.

Herpes

This pathology is caused by a common infection. It appears when the immune system is under stress. Simple herpes and herpes zoster (St. Anthony's fire) are cured by using Aloe arborescens-based products because of their antibacterial, antiviral, anti-inflammatory and immunomodulatorial properties.

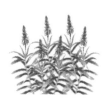

Chemotherapy-Related Weakening of the Body

Aloe arborescens' biological potential is also effective in relieving the debilitating effects of chemotherapy used to treat cancer. Immune system stimulation and proper functioning strengthen the body in regaining physical and psychological well being after chemotherapy-related aftereffects.

Psoriasis

A specific cure for psoriasis does not exist in medicine today. This pathology can be controlled by using Aloe arborescens as a topical treatment.

Respiratory System

Chronic or acute inflammatory manifestations commonly found in influenza and bacterial infections are effectively treated by Aloe arborescens. The use of this plant is effective in the following cases:

Laryngitis and Bronchitis

Pure Aloe-based inhalation can effectively fight against respiratory and bronchial infections. The acemannan makes this possible by activating the macrophage and lymphocytes immune defense against infection. The solution to this problem is also attained by vegetable sterol antiflogistic and lenitive actions.

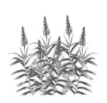

Riniti and Tonsillitis

The germicidal actions of some anthraquinones prove to be a valid remedy for these issues.

In concluding this rapid presentation of the healthy and therapeutic uses of the Aloe plant, it should be repeated that the versatility of this plant on numerous different pathologies afflicting the human body is endless. It is noted that, in general pharmaceutical preparation, only one pharmaceutical factor is capable in counteracting a specific pathology. This is not the case for Aloe. Aloe provides numerous herbal therapeutic factors that interact individually or together to positively counteract various pathologies. This can be seen in the following bibliographical pages.

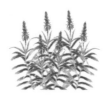

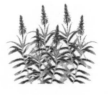

Bibliography, including Specific International Journals

Acevedo-Duncan, M., Russell, C., Patel, S., Patel, R.: Aloe-emodin-modulates PKC isozymes, inhibits proliferation, and induces apoptosis in U-373MG glioma cella. International Immuno-pharmacology 4(14):1775-1784., 2004.

Afzal, M., Ali, M., Hassan, R.A.H., Sweedan, N., Dhami, M.S.I.: Identification of some prostanoids in Aloe vera extracts. Planta Medica 57, 38-40, 1991.

Ando, N., Yamaguchi, I.: Sitosterol from Aloe vera gel. Kenkyu Kiyo-Tokyo Kasei Daigaku 30, 1520, 1990.

Anton, R., Haag-Berrurier, M.: Therapeutic use of natural anthra-quinone for other than laxative actions. Pharmacology 20, 104-112, 1980.

Ashley, F.L, O'Loughlin, B.J., Peterson, R., Fernandez, L., Stein, H., Schwartz, A.N.: The use of Aloe vera in the treatment of thermal and irradiation burns in laboratory animals and humans. Plastic and Reconstructive Surgery 20, 383-396, 1957.

Avila, H., Rivero, J., Herrera, F., Fraile, G.: Cytotoxicity of a low molecular weight fraction from Aloe vera (Aloe barbadensis Miller) gel. Toxicon 35, 1423-1430, 1997.

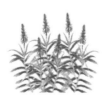

Azghani, A.O., Williams, I., Holiday, D.B., Johnson, A.R.: A betalinked mannan inhibits adherence of Pseudomonas aeruginosa to human lung epithelial cells. Glycobiology 5, 39-44, 1995.

Basso, G., Diaspro, A., Salvato, B., Carli, M., Palu, G.: Aloe-emodin is a new type of anticancer agent with selective activity against neuroectodermal tumors. Cancer Research 60(11):2800-2804, 2000.

Beppu, H., Koitz, T., Shimpo, K., Chihara, T., Hoshino, M., Ida, C., Kuzuya, H.: Radical-scavenging effect of Aloe arborescens Miller on prevention of pancreatic islet B-cell destruction in rats. Journal of Ethnopharmacology, 89 (1):27-45, 2003.

Beppu, H., Shimpo, K., Chihara, T., Kaneko, T., Tamai, I., Yamaji, S., Ozaki, S., Kuzuya, H., Sonoda, S.: Fujita Memorial Nanakuri Institute, Fujita Health University, 1865 Isshiki-cho, Hisai, Mie 514-1296, Japan. Anti-diabetic effects of dietary administration of Aloe arborescens Miller components on multiple low-dose streptozotocin-induced diabetes in mice: investigation on hypoglycemic action and systemic absorption dynamics of aloe components. J Ethnopharmacol. 103(3):468-77, 2006 Feb 20.

Bland, J.: Effect of orally consumed Aloe vera juice on gastrointestinal function in normal humans. Preventive Medicine 14, 152-154, 1985.

Blitz, J., Smith, J.W., Gerard, J.R.: Aloe vera gel in peptic ulcer therapy: preliminary report. Journal of the American Osteopathic Association 62, 731-735, 1963.

Bloomfield, F.: Miracle Plants: Aloe Vera. Century, London, 1985.

Brossat, J.Y., Ledeaut, J.Y., Ralamboranto, L., Rakotovao, L.H., Solar, S., Gueguen, A., Coulanges, P.: Immuno-stimulating properties of an extract isolated from Aloe vahombe. Archives Institut Pasteur Madagascar 48, 11-34, 1981.

Bruce, W.G.G.: Investigations of antibacterial activity in the Aloe. South African Medical Journal 41, 984, 1967.

Bruce, W.G.G.: Medicinal properties in the Aloe. Excelsa 57-68, 1975.

Capasso, F., Borrelli, F., Capasso, R., DiCarlo, G., Izzo, A.A., Pinto, L., Mascolo, N., Castaldo, S., Longo, R.: Aloe and its therapeutic use. Phytotherapy Research 12, S124-S127, 1998.

Cera, L.M., Heggers, J.P., Robson, M.C., Hagstrom, W.J.: The therapeutic efficacy of Aloe vera cream (Dermaide Aloe™) in thermal injuries. Two case reports. J. Am. Animal Hospital Assoc. 16, 768-772, 1980.

Coats, Bill C., R.Ph., C.C.N., with Ahola, Robert: Aloe Vera, the New Millennium, i Universe, 2003.

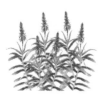

Danhof, Ivan E., M.D., Ph.D., (ND): The Fundamentals of Aloe Vera Mucopolysaccharides. Abstract: Dr. Danhof is regarded by many as the leading authority on the Aloe vera plant. This paper gives the fundamentals of how the polysaccharide molecules help the body in the healing process, 1994.

Danhof, Ivan E., M.D., Ph.D, (ND): Aloe Vera Leaf Handling and Constituent Variability; Remarkable Aloe – Aloe Through the Ages, Vol. 1, Omnimedicus Press, 1987.

Danhof, Ivan E, M.D., Ph.D.: Internal uses of Aloe vera. Abstract: Aloe used in intestinal disorders, atherosclerosis and coronary hearth disease, anti-cancer actions, immunity, 1988.

Danhof, Ivan E., M.D., Ph.D.: Aloe Vera, The Whole Leaf Advantage, 2000.

Davis, R.H.: Topical influence of Aloe vera on adjuvant arthritis, inflammation and wound healing. Physiologist 31, 206, 1988.

Davis, R.H., Agnew, P.S., Shapiro, E.: Anti-arthritic activity of anthraquinones found in Aloe for podiatric medicine. Journal of the American Podiatric Medical Association 76, 61-66, 1986.

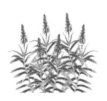

Davis, R.H., Kabbani, J.M., Maro, N.P.: Wound healing and anti-inflammatory activity of Aloe vera. Proceedings of the Pennsylvania Academy of Science 60, 79, 1986.

Davis, R.H., Leitner, M.G., Russo, J.: Topical anti-inflammatory activity of Aloe vera as measured by ear swelling. Journal of the American Podiatric Medical Association 77, 610-612, 1987.

Davis, R.H., Leitner, M.G., Russo, J.M., Byrne, M.E.: Anti-inflammatory activity of Aloe vera against a spectrum of irritants. Journal of the American Podiatric Medical Association 79, 263-276, 1989.

Davis, R.H., Maro, N.P.: Aloe vera and gibberellin. Anti-inflammatory activity in diabetes. Journal of the American Podiatric Medical Association 79, 24-26, 1989.

Davis, Robert H., Ph.D., Professour Emeritus of Physiology, Pennsylvania College of Podiatric Medicine: The Conductor-Orchestra Concept Of Aloe Vera, The Model For Aloe Vera.

Davis, Robert H., Ph.D.: Biological Activity of Aloe Vera.

Duke, J.A.: Aloe barbadensis Mill. (Liliaceae). CRC Handbook of Medicinal Herbs. CRC Press, Boca Raton, FL, pp. 31-32, 1985.

Egger, S., Brown, G.S., Kelsey, L.S., Yates, K.M., Rosenberg, L.J., Talmadge, J.E.: Hematopoietic augmentation by a beta-(1,4)-

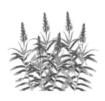

linked mannan. Cancer Immunology Immuno-therapy 43, 195-205, 1996.

Elkins, Rita, M.H.: Miracle Sugars, The Glyconutrient Link to Disease Prevention and Improved Health, Woodland Publishing, 2003

Finbar, Magee (Dr.): Health watch: Alternative path: Aloe, aloe what's all this then? The News Letter. Belfast, Northern Ireland. Abstract: Lists some of the benefits of Aloe and also some of the 75 plus nutritional substances. "What is also apparent is that the plant itself is better than the sum of the individual components. In some way the synergistic balance out performs isolated components." (2002, November 6).

Frumkin, A.: Aloe vera, salicylic acid and aspirin for burns. Plastic and Reconstructive Surgery 83, 196, 1989.

Fujita, K., Ito, S., Teradaira, R., Beppu, H.: Properties of a carboxypeptidase from Aloe. Biochemical Pharmacology 28, 1261-1262, 1979.

Fujita, K., Yamada, Y., Azuma, K., Hirozawa, S.: Effect of leaf extracts of Aloe arborescens Mill subsp. natalensis Berger on growth of Trichophyton entagrophytes. Anti-microbial Agents and Chemotherapy 35, 132-136, 1978.

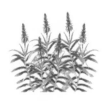

Furukawa, F., Nishikawa, A., Chihara, T., Shimpo, K., Beppu, H., Kuzuya, H., Lee, I.S., Hirosr, M.: Chemopreventive effects of <u>Aloe arborescens</u> on N-nitrosobis(2-oxopropyl) amine-induced pancreatic carcinogenesis in hamsters. Cancer Letters 178(2): 117-122, 2002.

Gardiner, T.: "Biological Activity of eight known dietary mono-saccharides required for glycoprotein synthesis and cellular recognition processes: summary," Glyco Science & Nutrition 1(13):1-4, 2000.

Gauntt, C., et al.: Aloe polymannose enhances anti-coxsackievirus antibody titres in mice, Phytotherapy Research, 14(4):261-6, 2000 June.

Gowda, D.C., Neelisiddaiah, B., Anjaneyalu, Y.V.: Structural studies of polysaccharides from Aloe vera. Carbohydrate Research 72, 201-205, 1979.

Grindlay, D., Reynolds, T.: The Aloe vera phenomenon: a review of the properties and modern uses of the leaf parenchyma gel. Journal of Ethnopharmacology 16, 117-151, 1986.

Haq, Q.N., Hannan, A.: Studies on glucogalactomannan from the leaves of Aloe vera, Tourn. (ex Linn.). Bangladesh Journal of Scientific and Industrial Research 16, 68-72, 1981.

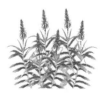

Heggers, J.P., Kucukcelibi, A., Listengarten, D., Stabenau, C.J., Ko, F., Broemeling, L.D., Robson, M.C., Winters, W.D.: Beneficial effect of Aloe on wound healing in an excisional wound model. Journal of Alternative and Complementary Medicine 2, 271-277, 1996.

Heggers, J.P., Pelley, R.P., Robson, M.C.: Beneficial effects of Aloe in wound healing. Phytotherapy Research 7, S48-S52, 1993.

Hiroko, Saito: Aloe's Effectiveness as an Anti-Inflammatory Agent, Department Of Pharmacy, Aichi Cancer Center, 1993

Hu, Y., Xu, J., Hu, Q.: Evaluation of antioxidant potential of aloe vera (Aloe barbadensis Miller) extracts. Journal of Agricultural and Food Chemistry 51(26):7788-7791, 2003.

Hutter, J.A., Salman, M., Stavinoha, W.B., Satsangi, N., Williams, R.F., Streeper, R.T., Weintraub, S.T.: Anti-inflammatory glucosyl chromone from Aloe barbadensis. Journal of Natural Products 59, 541-543, 1996.

Imanishi, K.: Aloctin A, an active substance of Aloe Arborescens Miller as an immunomodulator. Phytotherapy Research 7, S20-S22, 1993.

Jamieson, G.I.: Aloe vera (Aloe barbadensis Mill.). Queensland Agricultural Journal 110, 220, 1984.

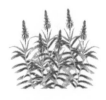

Kinoshita, K., Koyama, K., Takahashi, K., Noguchi, Y., Amano, M.: Steroid glucosides from Aloe barbadensis. Journal of Japanese Botany 71, 83-86, 1996.

Kodym, A.: The main chemical components contained in fresh leaves and in a dry extract from three years old <u>Aloe arborescens</u> Mill. grown in hothouses. Pharmazie 46, 217-219, 1991.

Kodym, A., Marcinkowski, A., Kukula, H., Department of Drug Form Technology, Ludwik Rydygier Medical University in Bydgoszcz: Technology of eye drops containing aloe (<u>Aloe arborescens</u> Mill.—Liliaceae) and eye drops containing both aloe and neomycin sulphate. Acta Poloniae Pharmaceutics. 60(1):31-9, 2003 Jan-Feb.

Koike, T., Beppu, H., Kuzuya, H., Maruta, K., Shimpo, K., Suzuki, M., Titani, K., Fujita, K.: A 35 kDa mannose-binding lectin with hemag-glutinating and mitogenic activities from 'Kidachi Aloe' (<u>Aloe arborescens</u> Miller var. natalensis Berger). Journal of Biochemistry 118, 1205-1210, 1995.

Koo, M.: Aloe vera: anticancer and antidiabetic effects. Phytother Res 8:461-4, 1994.

Kuo, P.L., Lin, T.C., Lin, C.C.: The antiproliferative activity of aloe-emodin is through p53-dependent and p21-dependent

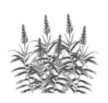

apoptotic pathway in human hepatoma cell lines. Life Sciences 71(16): 1879-1892, 2002.

Lee, K.H., Hong, H.S., Lee, C.H., Kim, G.A.: Induction of apoptosis in human leukaemic cell lines K562, HL 60 and U9337 by diethylhexylphthlatate isolated from Aloe vera Linne. Journal of Pharmacy and Pharmacology 52(8):1037-1041, 2000.

Lee, K.H., Klim, J.H., Liu, D.S., Kim, C.H.: Anti-leukaemic and anti-mutagenic effects of di(2-ethylhexyl)phthalate isolated from Aloe vera Linne. Journal of Pharmacy and Pharmacology 52(5):593-598, 2000.

Lefkowitz, D., et al.: "Effects of a glyconutrient on macrophage functions," International Journal of Immunopharmacology 22(4):299-308, 2000 Apr.

Leung, M.Y., Liu, C., Zhu, L.F., Hui, Y.Z., Yu, B., Fung, K.P.: Chemical and biological characterization of a polysaccharide biological response modifier from Aloe vera L. Glycobiology 14(6):501-5 10, 2004.

Lian, L.H., Park, E.J., Piao, H.S., Zhao, Y.Z., Soho, D.H.: Aloe-emodin-induced apoptosis in t-HSC/CI-6 cells involves a mitochondria-mediated pathway. Basic and Clinical Pharmacology and Toxicology 96(6):495-502, 2005.

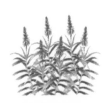

Lin, J.G., Chen, G.W., Li, T.M., Chouh, S.T., Tan, T.W., Chung, J.G.: Aloe-emodin induces apoptosis in T24 human bladder cancer cells through the p53-dependent apoptotic pathway. Journal of Urology 175(1):343-347, 2006.

Lindblad, W.J., Thul, J.: Sustained increase in collagen biosynthesis in acemannan impregnated PVA implants in the rat. Wound Repair and Regeneration 2, 84, 1994.

Lissoni Paolo, Rovelli Franco, Brivio Fernando, Zago Romano, Colciago Massimo, Messina Giuseppina, Mora Adelio, Porro Giorgio. A randomized study of chemotherapy versus biochemotherapy with chemotherapy plus Aloe arborescens in patients with metastatic cancer. Division of Radiation Oncology, St. Gerardo Hospital, Monza, Milan, Italy. p.lissoni@hsgerardo.org In Vivo 2009 Jan-Feb;23(1):171-5.

Liu, Y., Yang, H., Takatsuki, H., Sakanishi, A.: Effect of ultrasonic exposure of Ca++ -ATPase activity in plasma membrane from <u>Aloe arborescens</u> callus cells. Ultrasonic Sonochemistry 13(3):232-236, 2006.

McDaniel. H.R., Pulse, T.: Predition and Results Obtained Using Oral Acemannan in 41 Symptomatic HIV Patients. IV International Conference on Aids, Stockholm, Sweden, June 12-16, 1988.

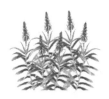

McDaniel, H. Reg., M.D.: Cancer, Is There A Role for Dietary Supplementation in Combination with Standard Cancer Therapy. Comprehensive Cancer Conference 2000, The Center for Mind-Body Medicine Washington, DC June 9-11, 2000 Sponsors: The University of Texas-Houston Medical School, The National Cancer Institute, The National Center for Complementary and Alternative Medicine, 2000.

McDaniel, H. Reg., M.D.: The Micronutrient Best Case Cancer Series: A Compendium of Medical Presentations Made at Cancer Conferences Between 2000 and 2004 documenting that the Quality of Life and Response to Standard Treatment Protocols for Malignancy Improved with Dietary Supplementation. These conferences included: The Comprehensive Cancer 2003 Conference held in Washington, D.C. and sponsored by the Center for Mind Body Medicine, National Cancer Institute, National Center for Complementary and Alternative Medicine of the National Institutes of Health, First International Conference for Integrative Oncology held in New York City, NY, in November 2004 and sponsored by the National Center for Complementary and Alternative Medicine of the National Institutes of Health and the Society for Integrative Oncology, 2000-2004.

McDaniel, H. Reg., M.D.: Hepatitis General Antiviral Activity is Supported by Glyconutrient Dietary Supplementation. Hepatitis Conference 2000 Miami Beach, Florida, June 3-4, 2000.

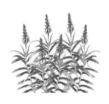

McDaniel, H. Reg., M.D.: AIDS Patient Responses Validate in Vitro Experiments Indicating Micronutrient Dietary Supplementation (DS) Supports Innate Antiviral Mechanisms and Restores Immune Function. 9th World Congress on Clinical Nutrition, The University of Westminster, London, England, June 24-26, 2002.

McDaniel, H. Reg., M.D.: The Molecular Biology of How Dietary Supplements Support Optimal Human Health, 2005.

McDaniel, H. Reg., M.D.: Lymphocyte Levels in Acemannan Treated HIV-1 Infected Long-Term Survivors, Abstract # PO-B29-2179, IXth International Conf. on AIDS, Berlin, 1993.

McDaniel, H. Reg., M.D.: The Source of the <u>Master</u> Glyconutrient.

Merzlyak, M., Solovchenko, A., Pogosyan, S.: Department of Physiology of Microorganisms, Faculty of Biology, Moscow State University, 1 19992, GSP-2, Moscow, Russia. mnm@6. Celllmm.bio.msu.ru Optical properties of rhodoxanthin accumulated in <u>Aloe arborescens</u> Mill. Leaves under highlight stress with special reference to its photoprotective function. Photochemical & Photobiological Sciences. 4(4):333-40, 2005 Apr.

Morita, H.; Mizuuchi, Y.; Abe, T.; Kohno, T.; Noguchi, H.; Abe, I.: Institution Mitsubishi Kagaku Institute of Life Sciences (MITILS). Cloning and functional analysis of novel aldo-keto

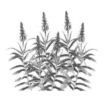

reductase from <u>Aloe arborescens.</u> Biological 8, Pharmaceutical Bulletin. 30 (12):2262-7, 2007 Dec.

Nacci, Giuseppe., M.D. Thousand Plants Against Cancer without Chemo-Therapy, Chapter 9.b: Aloe Aborescens October 2008

Obata, M., Ito, S., Beppu, H., Fujita, K., Nagatsu, T.: Mechanism of anti-inflammatory and antithermal burn action of Aloe arborescens Miller var. Natalensis Berger. Phytotherapy Research 7, s30-s33, 1993.

Parish, Christopher R.: Innate Immune Mechanisms: Nonself Recognition, Australian National University, Canberra, Australia, July 1999.

Pecere, T., Gazzolz, M.V., Mucignat, C., Paralin, C., Vecchia, F. D., Cavaggioni, A., Pierce, R.F.: Comparison between the nutritional contents of the Aloe gel from conventionally and hydroponically grown plants. Erde International 1, 37-38, 1983.

Pecere, T., Gazzolz, M.V., Mucignat, C., Paralin, C., Vecchia, F. D., Cavaggioni, A., Basso, G., Diaspro, A., Salvato, B., Carli, M., Palu, G.: Aloe-emodin is a new type of anticancer agent with selective activity against neuroectodermal tumors. Cancer research 60 (11):2800-2804, 2000.

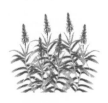

Peuser, Michael: Capillaries Determine Our Fate/Aloe Empress of the Medical Plants, by St. Hubertus Produtos Naturals Ltda. Brazil: 91-101, 2003.

Pittman, J.C.: Immune-Enhancing Effects of Aloe, Health Conscious, 13(1) 28-30, 1992.

Plaskett, Lawrance G. (BA, PhD, CChem, FRIC): Aloe vera and the human immune system. *Aloe Vera Information Services* (newsletter). Camelford, Cornwall, UK: Biomedical Information Services Ltd. Abstract: Specialized molecules in Aloe vera whole leaf extract interact with some special "receptor" substances that are embedded into the outer membrane of our immune system cells. The result is that the immune system cells are galvanized into action. In particular, the class of cells known as "phagocytes" increase the activities by which they attack and then engulf bacteria, waste products and debris. This increase in scavenging activities cleanses and protects the body, with knock-on benefits for a whole cascade of different medical conditions. The literature indicates that a common mechanism in this respect probably exists in both humans and animals and that both can benefit enormously from the use of Aloe vera, 1996, April.

Plaskett, Lawrance G. (BA, PhD, CChem, FRIC): Aloe vera and cancer. Aloe Vera Information Services (newsletter). Camel-

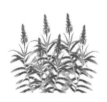

ford, Cornwall, UK: Biomedical Information Services Ltd., 1996, September.

Plaskett, Lawrance, BA, PhD, CChem, FRIC: Aloe Vera, Aloe In Alternative Medicine Practice.

Plaskett, Lawrance G. (BA, PhD, CChem, FRIC): The healing properties of Aloe. *Aloe Vera Information Services* (newsletter). Camelford, Cornwall, UK: Biomedical Information Services Ltd., 1996, July.

Pugh, N., Ross, S.A., El Sohly, M.A., Pasca, D.S.: Characterization of *Aloeride, a new high-molecular weight polysaccharide from Aloe vera with potent immuno-stimulatory activity. Journal of Agricultural and Food Chemistry 49(2): 1030-1034, 2001.

Pulse, T.L. (MD), & Uhlig, Elizabeth (RRA): A significant improvement in a clinical pilot study utilizing nutritional supplements, essential fatty acids and stabilized Aloe vera juice in 29 HIV seropositive, ARC and AIDS patients. Journal of Advancement in Medicine, 3(4), 1990, Winter.

Qiu, Z., Jones, K., Wylie, M., Jia, G., Orndoref, S.: Modified Aloe barbadensis polysaccharide with immuno-regulating activity. Planta Medica 66(2): 152-156, 2000.

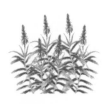

Reynolds, T., Dweck, A. C.: Aloe vera leaf gel: a review update. Journal of Ethnopharmacology. 68, 3-37, 1999.

Ross, S.A., El Sohly, M.A., Wilkins, S.P.: Quantitative analysis of Aloe vera mucilagenous polysaccharides in commercial Aloe vera products. Journal of AOAC International 80, 455-457, 1997.

Rubel, B.L.: Possible mechanisms of the healing actions of Aloe gel. Cosmetics and Toiletries 98, 109-114, 1983.

Sabeh, F., Wright, T., Norton, S.J.: Isozymes of superoxide dismutase from Aloe vera. Enzyme Protein 49, 212-221, 1996.

Saito, H.: Purification of active substances of <u>Aloe arborescens</u> Miller and their biological and pharmacological activity. Phytotherapy Research 7, S14-S19, 1993.

Sampedro, M.C., Artola, R.L., Murature, M., Murature, D., Ditamo, Y., Roth, G.A., Kivatinitz, S.: Mannan from Aloe saponaria inhibits tumoral cell activation and proliferation. International Immuno-pharmacology 4(3):4 1 1-4 18, 2004.

Saoo, K., Miki, H., Ohmori, M., Winters, W.D.: Antiviral activity of Aloe extracts against cytomegalovirus. Phytotherapy Research 10, 348-350, 1996.

Schechter, S.R.: Aloe vera: the healing plant. Health Foods Business, 23-24, 1994.

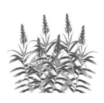

Shelton, R.M.: Aloe vera: Its chemical and therapeutic properties. International Journal of Dermatology 30, 679-683, 1991.

Shida, T., Yagi, A., Nishimura, H., Nishioka, I.: Effect of Aloe extract on peripheral phagocytosis in adult bronchial asthma. Planta medica 51, 273-275, 1985.

Shimpo, K., Beppu, H., Chihara, T., Kaneko, T., Shinzato, M., Sonoda, S.: Fujita Memorial Nanakuri Institute, Fujita Health University, Tsu, 1865 Isshiki-cho, Hisai Mie 514-1296 Japan. Effects of Aloe arborescens ingestion on azoxymethane-induced intestinal carcinogenesis and hematological and bio-chemical parameters of male F344 rats. Asian Pacific Journal of Cancer Prevention: Apjcp. 7(4):585-90, 2006 Oct-Dec.

Shimpo, K., Chihara, T., Beppu, H., Ida, C., Kaneko, T., Nagatsu, T., Kuzuya, H.: Inhibition of azoxymethane-induced aberrant crypt foci formation in rat colorectum by whole leaf Aloe arborescens Miller, var. natalensis Berger. Phytotherapy Research 15(8):705-711, 2001.

Shimpo, K., Ida, C., Chihara, T., Beppu, H., Kaneko, T., Kuzuya, H.: Aloe arborescens extract inhibits TPA-induced ear oedema, putrescine increase and tumour promotion in mouse skin. Phytotherapy Research 16(5):491-493, 2002.

Shimpo, K., Chihara, T., Beppu, H., Ida, C., Kaneko, T., Hoshino, M., Kuzuya, H.: Inhibition of azoxymethane-induced DNA

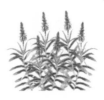

adduct formation by <u>Aloe arborescens</u> var. natalensis. Asian Pacific Journal of Cancer Prevention 4(3):247-251, 2003.

Siegel, Dr. R., M.D.: Aloe, Immunity and Health CareScience papers presented to the Annual International Environmental Conference, 1998.

Siegel, Dr. R., M.D.: The Science of Immunity/ The Regulation of Immunity

Siegel, Dr. R., M.D.: Natural Plant Molecules

Soeda, M., Otomo, M., Ome, M., Kawashima, K.: Studies on antibacterial and anti-fungal activity of Cape Aloe. Nippon Saikingaku Zasshi 21, 609-614, 1966.

Stuart, R.W., Lefkowitz, D.L., Lincoln, J.A., Howard, K., Gelderman, M.P., Lefkowitz, S.S.: Upregulation of phagocytosis and candicidal activity of macrophages exposed to the immunostimulant, acemannan. International Journal of Immunopharmacology 19, 75-82, 1997.

Sydiskis, R.J., Owen, D.G., Lohr, J.L., Rosler, K.H., Blomster, R.N.: Inactivation of enveloped viruses by anthraquinones extracted from plants. Antimicrobial Agents and Chemotherapy 35, 2463-2466, 1991.

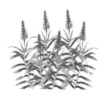

Syed, T.A., Ahmad, A., Holt, A.H., Ahmad, S.A., Ahmad, S.H., Afzal, M.: Management of psoriasis with Aloe vera extract in a hydrophilic cream: a placebo-controlled, double blind study. Tropical Medicine and International Health 1, 505-509, 1996.

T'Hart, L.A., Nibbering, P.H., van den Barselaar, M.T., van Dijk, H., van den Berg, A.J., Labadie, R.P.: Effects of low molecular constituents from Aloe vera gel on oxidative metabolism and cytotoxic and bactericidal activities of human neutrophils. International Journal for Immunophar-macology 12, 427-434, 1990.

T'Hart, L.A., van den Berg, A. J. J., Kuis, L., van Dijk, H., Labadie, R.P.: An anticomplementary polysaccharide with immuno-logical adjuvant activity from the leaf parenchyma gel of Aloe vera. Planta Medica 55, 509-512, 1989.

T'Hart, L.A., van Enckevort, P.H., van Dijk, H., Zaat, R., de Silva, K.T.D., Labadie, R.P.: Two functionally and chemically distinct immunomodulatory compounds in the gel of Aloe vera. Journal of Ethnopharmacology 23, 61-71, 1988.

Tanaka, M., Misawa, E., Ito, Y., Habara, N., Nomaguchi, K., Yamada, M., Toida, T., Hayasawa, H., Takase, M., Inagaki, M., Higuchi, R., Biochemical Research Laboratory, Morinaga Milk Industry Co., Ltd, Kanagawa, Japan: Identification of five

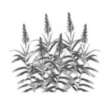

phytosterols from Aloe vera gel as anti-diabetic com-pounds. Biological 8, Pharmaceutical Bulletin. 29(7):1418-22, 2006 Jul.

Teradaira, R., Shinzato, M., Beppu, H., Fujita, K.: Antigastric ulcer effects of <u>Aloe arborescens</u> Mill. var. natalensis Berger. Phyto-therapy Research 7, S34-S36, 1993.

Tizard, I., Carpenter, R.H., Kemp, M.: Immunoregulatory effects of a cytokine release enhancer (Acemannan). International Congress of Phytotherapy, 1991, Seoul, Korea, 68, 1991.

Tizard Ian R., BVMS, PhD, Carpenter Robert H., DVM, MS, McAnalley Bill H., PhD and Kemp Maurice C.: The biological activities of mannans and related complex carbohydrates. Department of Veterinary Microbiology and Parasitology, College of Veterinary Medicine. Texas A&M University, College Station, TX, and Carrington Laboratories, Inc. Irving, TX, USA August 21, 1989.

Wang, Z.W., Zhopu, J.M., Huang, Z.S., Yang, A.P., Liu, Z.L., Xia, Y.F., Zeng, Y.X., Zhu, X.F.: Aloe polysaccharide mediated radio-protective effect through the inhibition of apoptosis. Journal of Radiation Research (Tokyo) 45(3):447-454, 2004.

Wasserman, L., Avigad, S., Berry, E., Nordenberg, J., Fenig, E.: The effect of aloe-emodin on the proliferation of a new merkel carcinoma cell line. American Journal of Dermato-pathology 24(1): 17-22, 2002.

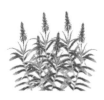

Wickline, M.M.: Prevention and treatment of acute radiation dermatitis: a literature review. Oncology Nursing Forum 3 1(2):237-247, 2004.

Willner, Robert E., M.D., Ph.D.: Whole Leaf Aloe Vera: The Cancer Solution, Peltec Publishing Co., Inc., 1994.

Winters, Wendell D.: Aloe Medicinal Substances Present And Future Potentials, Associate Professor of Microbiology Director, Phytobiology Studies Program, University of Texas Health Science Center, Polypeptides of Aloe barbadensis Miller., Phytotherapy Research, February, 2006.

Wozniewski, T., Blaschek, W., Franz, G.: Isolation and structure analysis of a glucomannan from the leaves of Aloe arborescens var. Miller. Carbohydrate Research 198, 387-391, 1990.

Yagi, A., Harada, N., Shimomura, K., Nishioka, I.: Bradykinin-degrading glycoprotein in Aloe arborescens var. natalensis. Planta Medica 53, 19-21, 1987.

Yagi, A., Harada, N., Yamada, H., Iwadare, S., Nishioka, I.: Anti-bradykinin active material in Aloe saponaria. Journal of Pharmaceutical Sciences 71, 1172-1174, 1982.

Yagi, A., Shida, T., Nishimura, H.: Effect of amino acids in Aloe extract on phagocytosis by peripheral neutrophil in adult

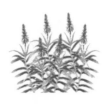

bronchial asthma. Japanese Journal of Allergology 36, 1094-1101, 1987.

Yamamoto, M., Masui, T., Sugiyama, K., Yokota, M., Nakagomi, K., Nakazawa, H.: Anti-inflammatory active constituents of <u>Aloe arborescens</u> Miller. Agricultural and Biological Chemistry 55, 1627-1629, 1991.

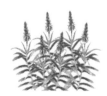

INDEX

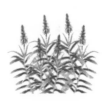

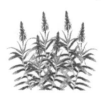

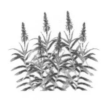